Corporealities: Discourses of Disability

David T. Mitchell and Sharon L. Snyder, editors

Points of Contact

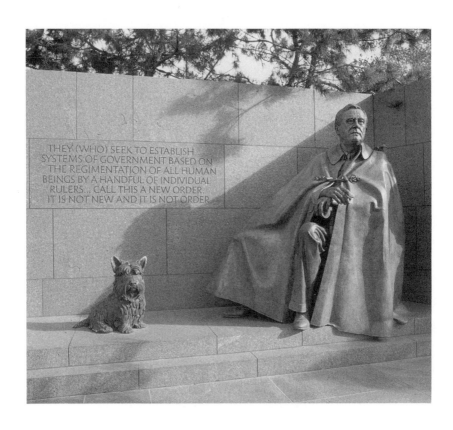

Franklin Delano Roosevelt and Fala, bronze sculpture by Neil Estern,
Franklin Delano Roosevelt Memorial.
Photo by Terry Adams, National Park Service.

Points of Contact

DISABILITY, ART, AND CULTURE

Susan Crutchfield and Marcy Epstein, Editors

Ann Arbor

THE UNIVERSITY OF MICHIGAN PRESS

Copyright © by the University of Michigan 2000
All rights reserved
Published in the United States of America by
The University of Michigan Press
Manufactured in the United States of America
∞ Printed on acid-free paper

2003   2002   2001   2000   4   3   2   1

A CIP catalog record for this book is available from the British Library.

Library of Congress Cataloging-in-Publication Data applied for
ISBN 0-472-09711-3 (cloth: alk. paper);
ISBN 0-472-06711-7 (pbk.: alk. paper)

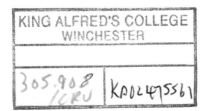

ACKNOWLEDGEMENTS

A number of people have provided us the invaluable support and fresh ideas that helped fuel this project over the last four years: Joanne Leonard, Harlan Hahn, Joseph Grigely, Simi Linton, Carrie Sandahl, Sharon Snyder, David Mitchell, Corbett O'Toole, Julie Amberg, Ruth Behar, Walter Harrison, Marvin Parnes, Paul Boylan, and Mary Higgins. We would also like to thank the artists, scholars, and activists who attended the This/Ability Conference and whose lives and work we wish to honor with our own. In particular, we acknowledge the planning committee that steered the conference: Hilary Cohen, Deena and Chris Baty, Daniel Jacobs, Lora Frankel, Julie Amberg, Sam Goodin, Brian Clapham, Ann Rockwell, Ron Sekulski, Sarah Innes, Lily Jarman-Rhode, Ron Yarrington, and Don Anderson.

Our special thanks to Larry Goldstein, for his wonderful sense of direction for this project in its first guise at *Michigan Quarterly Review* as well as for his encouragement in recreating the project in its present form. Our guest interns at *MQR*—Kirsten Kristofferson, John Morgan, Katerie Prior, Brian Walker, Leigh Lewis, and Inci Sayman—performed crucial research at several stages of the project. *MQR* administrative assistant Doris Knight deftly handled the office administration and follow-up. LeAnn Fields has been an expert guide and resource at the University of Michigan Press. We are grateful to our series editors, Sharon Snyder and David Mitchell, for their continuing support and advocacy.

Our families, partners, and friends have been indispensable to us.

Finally, we appreciate the chance to develop our teaching practice of disability texts and themes. For this we are indebted to our students and colleagues at the University of Michigan, Macalester College, the University of Wisconsin at LaCrosse, Henry Ford Community College, and The Roeper School.

NOTE TO TEACHERS AND STUDENTS

The works gathered here provide students multiple points of entry into the study of disability. There are pieces appropriate for the study of disability culture, disability art, disability identity, disability politics, disability as a minority experience within dominant culture, the disabled in contact with the nondisabled, and more. In addition to representing some of the foremost figures in the study of disability to date, our offerings in some cases include controversial voices for disability studies; they do not necessarily fall clearly into the current schema of disability art or criticism. This allows students to tread the path of controversy themselves, weighing possible meanings as well as their political and human implications. It is also an opportunity for teachers and students to discuss disability studies as an area of great significance in our culture, in the sense that it continues to evolve alongside and independently of academic or governmental bodies. There remains room for new ideas.

For example, Michael Downs's story "Rehearsal" provides students a scenario to discuss as one among many possible scripts for a relationship of care (and of husband and wife) when the receiver of care faces death. Does this script strip the cancer sufferer of her life too cavalierly, removing her importance from the story and lessening her presence in her husband's life even before she dies? Does this narrative offer an argument for assisted suicide—a scenario odious to disability activists for its suggestion that some lives are not worth living? Who is the story about? What alternate scripts can we imagine and rehearse? Other pieces invite investigation of the nature and scope of disability as a category of identity. Bell Gale Chevigny and Tobin Siebers ponder the personal costs and benefits of recognizing, and then accepting, the denial of ability as a key to their identities. Conversely, works by Sarah Ruden,

Sandra Gilbert, F. D. Reeve, and Reginald Shepherd challenge students to ponder whether the term *disability* can be stretched too thin and with what consequences. Are categories of disabled and nondisabled distinct? Perhaps more important, these and all of the other pieces in the collection offer myriad opportunities for understanding how disability permeates our individual lives as well as our collective social and artistic life.

While the volume spurs critiques from within a disability perspective, it also offers beauty, that is, the fundamental, diverse representation of aesthetics and values already at work in our collective culture. Furthermore, these works are interdisciplinary, giving introductory and upper-level students an approach to disability studies that is accessible across the vocabularies of individual disciplines. Students will want to study these pieces as contributions not only to disability studies and culture but also to their secondary fields: performance studies, art and art history, medicine, philosophy, political science, cultural studies, American studies, film and video studies, literature, creative writing, women's studies, and poetry. Teachers will want to consider including selections from this volume in syllabi for courses in the various departments and disciplines that contribute to disability studies.

It is our intention that, by considering these pieces, students might come to their own conclusions about the cohesion and diversity of disability culture. Consider the point of such contact: we hope that conversations among readers of all stripes will generate new questions about the ideological terrain of culture as well as the transformations such queries bring.

CONTENTS

SUSAN CRUTCHFIELD AND MARCY EPSTEIN

INTRODUCTION

Several events of the past few years have turned disability and disability "culture" into a cause célèbre of intellectuals, artists, civil rights activists, and others. News of preliminary plans for a national Mall memorial of Franklin Delano Roosevelt spurred a controversy between its designers and the members of Americans Disabled for Attendant Programs Today (ADAPT); the political long arm of the disability community demanded truth in representation, truth in art, truth about disability. Under contention was the memorial's depiction of the president without his wheelchair or crutches, an image that the designers argued was true to FDR's public depiction of himself and that ADAPT argued was simply untrue. Another controversy over disability representation pitted Disney Studios against the National Federation of the Blind (NFB); Disney's plans to release a live-action film version of the profoundly nearsighted Mr. Magoo cartoon elicited censure from the NFB, who felt the cartoon-dolt-turned-real-life-fool trafficked in harmful stereotypes of the vision impaired. The NFB lost its battle to stop production of the film. Pro golfer Casey Martin, who has a severe congenital disability affecting one leg, won the right in a lawsuit against the PGA to use a cart on the PGA and Nike tours. On a lighter note, Mattel's Barbie welcomed Share a Smile Becky (with wheelchair accessory) to her plastic and paint community. And, uniting fact with fiction, the nation's fictional superhero transmogrified into human proportions as Christopher Reeve leapt over the edifices of ablism and quadriplegic injury into the imaginations of mainstream America; he has become a screen director and national spokesman for spinal cord injury research.

While disability has gained public and academic attention from these events and from the aftereffects of the Americans

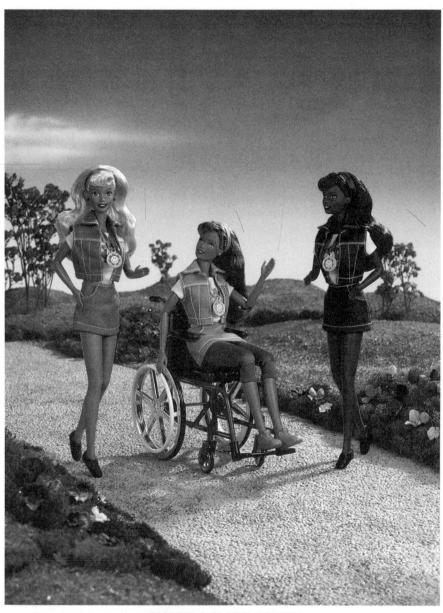

SHARE A SMILE BECKY

In conjunction with The National Parent Network on Disabilities, Mattel, Inc. developed the first 11½ inch fashion doll that comes with her own wheelchair. "The Share a Smile line of dolls includes Share a Smile Barbie and Share a Smile Christie, an African-American friend to Barbie and Becky, each in coordinating denim outfits and friendship necklaces."

with Disabilities Act, questions of disability representation, access, and identity remain. This area of inquiry constitutes the "undiscovered" territory of the late twentieth century. We write "undiscovered" with a note of irony, since these questions have been broached by disabled people since the beginning of time. Nonetheless, multiculturalism has signaled an end to the proprietariness of art and culture and even of the selfhood that has long eluded many disabled people. In its place is the topic *disability* and, with it, a sense that Deaf and disabled people possess the power to be self-determining. This sensibility provides a legitimate context in which to create art, literature, and scholarship that account for their/our existence and to make culture, the American way, in their/our image. This collection of essays, poems, and stories offers an assessment of disability as an aesthetic, political, and cultural idea. Disability "cultures" (including those that reject the *disabled* adjective, such as some members of deaf and blind communities) have existed in the past but have not been named. In our culture disability, like art, has no particular physical geography, though history has treated the category as something manifest, palpable, boundaried. Until recently, we have had few intellectual spaces in which activists, scholars, and artists could investigate the breadth and scope of disabled experience and representation. It is at the present, formative moment in the cultural history of deafness and disability that the works in this volume take up their collective artistic and scholarly tasks.

When this project began, in 1995, we felt there were few compelling collections of writings that discussed disability in the humanities in a manner that did not continue to pathologize or infantilize disability as a medical condition. Yet in the intervening years several scholars, activists, and artists have burst into mainstream academia with texts that follow historian Paul Longmore's injunction to shift our understanding of disability away from a medical model and toward that of a cultural "minority." Rosemarie Garland Thomson, Lennard Davis, Anne Finger, Sharon Snyder and David Mitchell, Simi Linton, Ann Pointon and Chris Davies, Kenny Fries, Adrienne Asch, Susan Wendell, Shelley Tremain, Brenda Bruegemann, Paul Longmore, David Hevey, Nicholas Mirzoeff, Michael Berubé, and others have emerged as powerful public and academic voices in the new "field(s)" of disability studies.

Such a designation as *field* has sparked a tremendous interest at all institutional levels as well. The Modern Language Association's (MLA's) permanent Committee on Disability Issues recently appointed Thomson as the first self-identified disabled person to sit on the MLA Task Force on Campus Bigotry, and the MLA has recognized a Disability Studies Discussion Group to ensure representation of existing and new scholarship in the field from year to year. The American Studies Association now includes a Disability Studies in the Humanities Subject Platform within its Crossroads Project; the Publications of the Modern Language Association (PMLA) now carries a disability bibliography. All of these developments have brought renewed and broader attention to the journal of the Society for Disability Studies, *Disability Studies Quarterly*, as well as the society's annual multidisciplinary conference. Longmore and Carol Gill have received a major grant to pursue projects on disability, curriculum, and social science. The field has quickly blossomed among promising interdisciplinary concentrations at the Universities of Hawaii, New Hampshire, Illinois at Chicago, and at Syracuse University, among others. Even inter-institutional developments in disability studies in the humanities have become a reality; the Disability Studies in the Humanities listserve (DS-HUM@LISTSERV.GEORGETOWN.EDU), currently administered by Martha Stoddard Holmes, links scholars with and without university affiliation in conversations about defining disability, new texts and institutional issues, course syllabi in disability studies, and more.

To call this explosion of scholarship the birth of a new discipline, however, would be palliative and perhaps a misnomer. People with disabilities are still subject to discriminatory practices that eat up the creative energies necessary to write about disability critically, or expressively, in an academy finally more open to hearing about disability folks than about where to put the ramp or hire the interpreter. Such works emerging in this climate, while ambitious and compelling, are nonetheless first forays into an intellectual miasma of the shifting terms, tattered history, and impenetrable swell of the culture that forms the context for such work. With respect to disability, the amnesia of our collective past is too profound to theorize at a glance. The various players, programs, and ideas that compose the picture of disability to date could, without further investigation and innovation, lead to a vast oversimplification of disability in definition, practice, and expression. Consequently, we have been interested in the "points of contact" among disability cultures as these emerge as well as those between disability culture and the status quo, the culture busily being remapped with markers of disability representation.

The University of Michigan's This/Ability interdisciplinary conference on disability and the arts, which we coordinated with Joanne Leonard in the spring of 1995, represented only the second time a conference was dedicated to themes of disabilities and the humanities and the first time that national disability activists, scholars, and artists assembled to discuss disability in the academy and in its relationship to the arts. Since then, we have grown increasingly aware of the impact of this conference, for better and for worse. Accommodation problems we experienced at the conference and at its art exhibit, "Vis/Ability: Views from the Interior," became symbolic of the dangers of nondisabled and institutional participation in the disability movement within the academy. On the other hand, we have received numerous reports of creative projects and scholarly partnerships that the conference helped forge across subcultures (both disciplinary and related to disability). Part of the problem, and its solution, was the recognition among participants that we were practicing a relatively new discipline and experiencing a complex political struggle over the identity of people attached to its development; however, the real trouble lay in blending academic and aesthetic concerns with the powerful notion of *culture*—in the "them and us" division that comes as we try to create a space for a disabled subject who has for centuries been the object of culture. As Snyder and Mitchell explore in *Vital Signs*—their video documentary of the conference, which they discuss in the essay "Talking about *Talking Back*"—this intention to be in control of words, ideas, and images is a main goal of creating disability culture. As their essay implies, many of us, disabled and nondisabled, tread new territories while evaluating and enforcing preexisting models of identity politics and disability "authority"—a mix of messages about scholarly production both insightful and inciteful.

That conference documented the need for further exploration, as this collection and its title shows. Whereas defining disability was not as much the point of the conference as exploring the ways we represent it, we still require definitions. Reflecting the fact that there can be no one defining disability, this collection includes contributors who speak to the far-reaching social and personal effects of acculturating disability from margin to center. Such a category of disability includes a spectrum of descriptors: access, blindness, mobility, the Deaf, environmental sensitivity, prosthetics, the freak, developmental disabilities, aging, AIDS, the patient, eugenics, illness, body standards, the villain, eating disorders, paralysis, class, attendant care, gender, sexuality, wounding, the poster child, language, the senses, and more. The included works demonstrate the compelling subject of disability in cultural studies and art—the dimension that disability adds to feminist and postcolonial critique, for example—while continuing to document the breadth of concrete experiences that already define the minority model of disability and its institutional response.

Describing his process of rehabilitation after polio as a "falling into life," Leonard Kriegel seeks a doctrine that "strips away the spiritual mumbo jumbo and the procrustean weight of existential anxiety."[1] This falling, warns Kriegel, is not a metaphor but a close description of the social process of living with a disability. The metaphorical use of disability angers many artists and scholars in disability studies when it misdescribes or even denies the reality of what it means to be disabled. Several of our authors take up this issue directly. Carol Poore discusses how media images of Germany's wheelchair-using politician Wolfgang Schäuble swing between representing his chair as "a fact of his life" and as an ominous image of the "disturbance and disruption of the well-ordered, normative physical world." Victoria Ann Lewis critiques the remarkable flexibility of disability as a trope of humanity, juxtaposing Richard III—one of theater's best-known villains whose dark psyche is made manifest on his crippled body—with Tiny Tim, "who manifests innocence and goodness in the world." But metaphors can be powerfully productive, too. They draw linguistic alliances; they break them. Metaphor expresses perspective and is, by extension, a document of voice and subjectivity. Like Marko's wheelchair in Susan Fernbach's poem "Wheelchair," a metaphor is, for representing disability, both "a carrot, and a stick."

Along with *how,* the issue of what and who defines and represents disability in our culture continues to be a highly charged debate, one that must continue for a long time. As we live every day of our lives in America, those who are disabled think "we" know who "we" are and who "they" are. "They," after all, know who "they" are: dominant culture assumes an able body. Unlike the stable dyads of early feminism and civil rights—the he's and she's, whites and blacks—the logos of disability enters politics in highly dynamic forms. Wheelchairs, canes, and walkers are visible markers of disability. Aches and pains, scars, poverty and immobility, political silence, discrimination, cruelty from others, and dependence mark disability. This territory is marked for a reason. Extending disability past the concrete experience of disabled individuals risks the well-being, and the ire, of our incipient, collective "disabled" community. In our search for contributors we kept this in mind, wanting the voices of disabled writers and artists to represent themselves and to make direct contact with readers.

Situations of contact—including the Michigan conference, the 1994 Chautauqua of the Mark Taper Forum, the Theater and Disability Conference in Britain in 1992, and the Society for Disability Studies—make at least three things perfectly clear: disability is about lives; there is an art to living and showing disability; and disability is political. A great expanse of our culture has already been inflected with disability art and scholarship, just not *marked* as such. For many, even a primary metaphor of identity, *the person as disabled,* is only recently safe to claim. Bell Gale Chevigny, writing of her training with Joe Chaikin during the 1994 Disability Project at the Public Theater in New York, is surprised to employ the syllogism *disabled* for herself as she begins to practice with other disabled and nondisabled actors. Yet Chevigny finds the term continuously useful as a way to acknowledge and accept her weakening body as it probes and invents the field of representation around it and Chaikin's company. Tracing the theater project with graceful strokes through the lives of its disabled actors and its moments of progress, she queries the history written on disabled bodies, the "blank slates" of Able Bodies, and the irony of evolution that comes with her particular sort of consciousness, a disabled consciousness: "we see their fear of mortality and terror of dependency, heightened in a culture that equates loss of self-reliance with death. We are an enviable vanguard, but a vanguard nonetheless."

Does Chevigny's vanguard represent a viable disability art, and does a disabled consciousness of art know its bounds? Is this consciousness reserved for those who experience disability in their everyday lives? Is this what makes disabled people different from nondisabled people and disability art and culture different for that evolution? Chevigny sets out such useful questions: "Can our changed state—once we have accepted it—give us superior appreciation of vulnerability and interdependence? Can we re-vision our relationship with the others? Are we deficient, or they, because we know the body's secret destiny that they shrink from? Are we their spooks?" How to break through what Chevigny calls the "mutually crippling hierarchy" of a culture with its lines of ability and disability drawn remains one of the pressing questions of disability in the theater and in the world it represents.

In contrast to this critical schema of identity, the disability experience comprises continuums of various individual experiences among other spectrums of difference and identity—notably those of race, class, and gender—that over the last few decades have recharged our national politics, universities, and art. In Joseph Grigely's unabridged version of "Postcards to Sophie Calle" the artist and critic discusses the use of art as a colonization of the blind while provocatively trading ideas of his own deafness and white maleness with those of violation and white femaleness, feminist and colonial interpretations of the gaze, and the meaning of touch. Along the way, Grigely raises crucial questions about form and method as well as content; in his search for "ambivalences" he suggests the powerful collectivity of a disabled minority that knows that, in the realm of representation, "each incursion made into their cultural territory is subject to critical veracity."

"Being" the figures who present this work, the guest editorial *we* also spans this range of identities, and we challenge our own veracity as part of a transformative disability study. We are both scholars, artists, and teachers. We have both experienced disabilities in our lifetimes and yet have at some point identified ourselves as "nondisabled"; we have purposely "outscribed" ourselves in the label but also are attracted to it, wary of how disability studies already suffers from the pangs of adolescent formulation. We entered this field for intellectual and ethical reasons. We are interested in the middle ground of disabled life, the experience of immersion, and in disability as a farrago of contradictory effects, a sideshow in which there is no outside. Between us we have been dependent and independent in turn, through depression, injury, chronic illness, and other disabling conditions. It is significant to us that *disability* describes a condition that rests both in identity and in a complex set of social relations that can affect many people, if not all, and all sentient life.

Depicting the disability experience as one affecting many, if not all, does in a sense compete with another significant goal of disability studies: the legitimating and advancement of the disabled individual. Compiling this volume, we considered the implications of constructing a disability identity that fits a status quo; this would imply that disabled folks are mere nonselves waiting to become selves. Is the label *disability* a way to that self? At the risk of "confessional vulgarity" and a foul temper in "Staring at Yellow and Green (Life and Art and PMS)," Sarah Ruden seeks revelation about forms of disability that affect our lives in essential ways, chronically and behaviorally instead of visually or orally. Reflecting upon the convergence of her various identities—as a woman, as a sufferer of severe and often debilitating PMS, as an artist—Ruden self-consciously pushes the term *disabled* to its limits. In doing so, she raises important questions about the cultural inflections of femininity through disability as well as about the potential dangers—both personal and collective—of appropriating and misappropriating a disabled identity.

In some senses the territory of disability is extant, marked, and yet curiously invisible. Like Dallas Wiebe's critic-thief with Alzheimer's, it has lacked a name or an exhibit but not a presence. As Tobin Siebers explains, this region is the history of his life after polio, and it, like him, is his "withered limb," the limbic extension of his identity through the part of himself that is himself. In the context of this volume Sandra Gilbert's memoir of her deceased husband claims disability as a metaphor of loss, but at the same time it records a very real debility: her loss is like a phantom made material again via electronic mail, the prosthetic extension of self in the cyber age. Among our poems, too, lie these less penetrable territories, areas where our disabilities and abilities coalesce so closely as to loosen the definitions of each completely from human bodies. Burton Raffel's rose curls and clings, "clearly bursting backward into existence / somewhere behind my blindness." These are not dismissive metaphors of disability: Gilbert's "unseen folds" and Reginald Shepherd's broken Eros enable the tough tread from one constellation of identity to another. These are expressions—beautiful, freakish expressions—of the struggle of individuals within a social hierarchy that marks disability as a sustained, permanent, and determining condition while forbidding them the comfort of their bodies or the bodies of their loved ones. As Willa Schneberg writes in her poem "Prothesis Maker," to "fling themselves / back into the family of the body" is to reclaim the emptied or withered places as habitations of people who feel belonging in the world.

Where, in our country, can such a symbolic, familial place be found? Next to mothers, but before apple pie, in the American psyche comes baseball. To the degree that sports bridge both art and popular imagination, baseball seems the most impenetrable and familiar of symbolic places, where the disabled figure dwindles away in a hospital bed in wait for a visit from Babe Ruth or Mickey Mantle. In Floyd Skloot's "Self-Portrait with 1911 NY Yankees Cap" the poem's diorama reverses its athletic personalities and its enervated spectators. As Skloot explains, his cap on his head after six years' illness, "The body is a machine / after all, and must fit its task." This credo fuels Joan Seliger Sidney's "Laps" as well, the image of her protagonist's athletic body "immobile in air" exemplary of the American drive. She writes of the machinery that runs the machine, the hydraulic chair, and an unknown swimmer who dresses the subject in the locker room. The physical triumph of body, will, and way—that which makes an athlete different from the weakling or wannabe—betrays the labor and effort of those who would join in the ranks, the family, the team, the nation. Susan Fernbach's endangered Marko, in "Wheelchair" (a portrait of Mark O'Brien, who was the subject of the Academy Award-winning documentary *Breathing Lessons* and who died this past summer), picks the right chair for the right body but lays it to rest when the perfect machine fails to ensure his safety in the world; it becomes a butler for his lover's clothes.

The social processes that condemn some and include others in the figurative ideals of society also shed light on the political and geographical terrains that have given form to history and its ideas of disability. The frontispiece image of FDR illustrates Carol Poore's investigation of how text, photograph, and political cartoon become the tools of creation, co-optation, and political fatalism for FDR as well as for wheelchair user Wolfgang Schäuble in his quest to succeed Helmut Kohl. Invoking past field conflicts, the day is "perfect . . . for imperfect bodies" in J. Quinn Brisben's account of a revered military cicerone, whose "elegant / Cane . . . blooms into a chair / For rest and close observation." The disabling of Civil War soldiers invokes for the poet a bygone wonderment and admiration that has in our time turned sour for veterans and other maimed people. Fleshing out our nation's lost history—the "bloody compounding of errors" before emancipation, which reduced the lives, circumstances, and sacrifices of the maimed to mere images of leftover bodies—Brisben reconstructs McClellan's career as a means to free a "future forever beyond our kenning." In the sense that the kenning is an ancient, epic form of identifying metaphor devoted to the exaltation of heroes, Brisben's poem takes back the term's power. The poet emphasizes the pride and belonging of the hero through a commingling of eras and battlegrounds, decrying the victim and giving disabled war vets their due. The land changes, the strategy changes, the human body changes, yet even in a reticent culture the sacred duty of giving one's leg or one's arm remains.

If athletes, politicians, and soldiers may be understood as special figures through which the personal territory of bodies extends into the public domain, then it is also possible that disability representation suggests the social sensibility that disabled individuals internalize as part of an everyday negotiation of the environment. We don't miss personal territory until we feel ourselves besieged with hostility, desire, freedom, or the frustration of impenetrable buildings, events, or relationships. Elizabeth Clare's tremors at a piano represent to her an experience more normal than "hands resting still as water." The assumption on the part of her curious observers that their bodies' movement is the simile for human nature provokes a curiosity of equal *forte:* the poet's own, palpable sense of the nondisabled "universe cradled inside," the one she has wondered about since her own birth with cerebral palsy. In contrast to Clare's sense of curiosity, Mark DeFoe jests over the enfeebled mall denizens of West Virginia who turn to gaze upon a young man who is not so much different from them as he is the epitome and embodiment of their region, values, and pace of life. "He comes to gibber, to remind / us that he is our kin." With his reproving yet affectionate gaze at all the Aunt Nevas, Cousin Clevises, and concordance sniffers at Walden's, DeFoe sketches how our curiosity for a man with a mental disability has outgrown our knowledge of the shared root of the human prime.

Such nondisabled voices as DeFoe's, as well as the relevance of the mainstream in creating "points of contact" between and among disabled cultures, makes it not only useful but also imperative to address the most expansive territory of the majority, that is, the nondisabled person's contact with disabled people and with themselves. Perhaps most compelling, since independence and dependence continue to be magnetic issues within the disability movement, is the figure of the caregiver. Stephen Dixon's story "The Motor Cart," for example, begins as a slow-motion action picture of a husband's attempts to restore the busted motor on his wife's cart but then turns to the mutual frustration, sensitivity, resignation, and need that accompany the eventualities of disabled life. In a world coded by identity politics, disability represents a politics, a contest of power over self-determination and cultural place; disability determines environment as much as it appears dependent upon it. Yet the most enabling factor in this environment are those delicate values—friendship and enmity, attention and neglect, love and hate, parenting and partnering, isolation, teaching, nursing, healing—that can be invoked and dismissed in a matter of moments by shifting perspectives.

With respect to disability and care, perhaps the most well-known demonstration of such values comes in the relationship between Anne Sullivan and Helen Keller. A paragon of inventive collaboration, their relationship becomes the stuff of literature, the curiosity of science, and the novelty of the theatrical world. Together Keller and Sullivan evoke the pith of the American imagination: success against adversity, freedom from dependence and for independence. Helen's so-called dependence on Anne is, understandably, the apparatus for the advancement of a fine mind. The extent of her disabilities attests to the achievement of her "normal" interactions. What Anne is to Helen, Helen is to a greater, collective culture, a Victorian America in search of its own artistic and cultural independence.

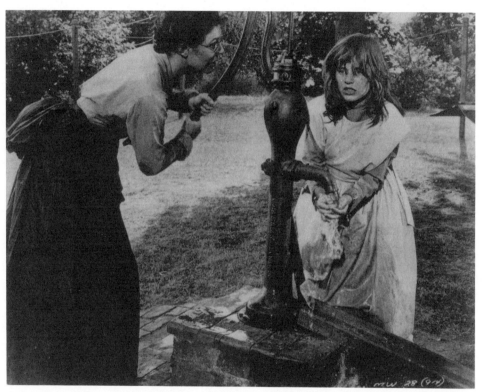

Anne Bancroft as Anne Sullivan with Patty Duke as Helen Keller in a scene from the film of William Gibson's play, *The Miracle Worker* (1962). Helen understands for the first time the connection between a word ("water") and the thing itself.

Thus in that era, and of monumental importance to this volume, a human being becomes, of necessity, the metonymy of an interdependent system: a prosthesis. Like Helen and Anne, all of us are natural and artificial necessities to each other, not equal, but in equilibrium, in authorship, social status, and ability; their autobiography is a sensational story of basic human connection. Through them we see that a human may be prosthetic when she is needed and that human relationships are dynamic in this respect. "Letters to Helen"—excerpted from Georgina Kleege's novel-in-progress—investigates a less uplifting moment in celebrity life, a time when the couple's success, their imagination even, was questioned over a matter of plagiarism when Keller was ten.

Kleege is a teacher of English and a blind woman, and thus her motive in describing the persecution of Keller seems at first the resurrection of the heroes and heroines of a newly born minority (although disabled people make up the largest minority in this country). The excerpt concludes with a narrative from the viewpoint of Mr. Anagnos, Sullivan's former mentor, which complicates the notions of creativity and difference already associated with Keller's persona as a gifted writer. Being a Greek immigrant whose place and importance within history are inextricably linked to those of Helen and Anne, Anagnos finds his own identity dependent upon them, both his students. He is as much outside of dominant American narratives as Helen is under question for her own. At the nexus of Anne and Helen's art and disability—and of Anagnos's social difference—emerges the social experience of interdependence. This representation of the treatment of disability is arguably a determining factor in how we construct the aesthetics and epistemes of humanity.

One of the most compelling myths of the caregiver is the dichotomy of patron saint and torturer, which revolves around the embodiment of necessary virtue, good intentions, pity, and protection, on the one hand, and judgment, abuse, and wrong intent, on the other. The media captures only the extremes of this split: the exemplary men and women who care for ill or crippled spouses or children against the tragic stories of dysfunction when a parent neglects a disabled child or a care attendant abuses an elderly client to death. Both extremes cultivate pity rather than care. Rarer are the stories of care that emphasize the respect for disabled people by the nondisabled. This respect is imperative and yet the most difficult point of contact to make. In its stead, the extremes of care draw attention because the middling nature of respecting individuals with the difference of disability remains well beyond the scope of our civilization at this time. Addressing the daily tribulations of living with disabled family members, F. D. Reeve considers the complex "association" of his nondisability with the disabilities of his wife, who is deaf, and his celebrity son, who faces a new personal identity as the nation's "fallen Superman."[2]

Robyn Sarah's essay, "Waiting for the Operation," also plays on an association between the mediated extremes of a poet in need and the mean of care. Her study of disability and resourcefulness begins with her own bitter struggle to take care of herself and then moves to Ken Hertz, a distant colleague whose "operation" she helps to finance. She discovers that Hertz has an aggressive system for dependent care, reliant on a complex composition of caregiving and corporate giving. On rigid schedules a nameless bevy of helpers ghostly and flawlessly tend to the so-called operation, enslaved yet inured to their client. Her story reminds us that disabled people can be educated consumers; for Sarah, Ken Hertz is also a consuming educator, his story fast overtaking her story. Given that Hertz is a spin doctor of his own condition, the essay ponders the next question: is the disabled figure at all *distinct* in a scenario of care? Michael Downs's short story "Rehearsal" offers a three-dimensional portrait of a troubled caregiver transfixed by both his wife's colon cancer and an opera, *The Inferno,* which he composes, dirge-like, in the months before her death. His wife grows increasingly indistinct in the blur of his divided attention, which devolves, it would seem, at her request. Downs's fiction wonders about faith—faith in living, faith in God, faith in marriage—and indeed we must take his wife's diminishing presence at the end of the story on faith as well. In death they do part. He is the caregiver who has been cared for too well: he has been cut loose, a composer without his muse.

The perversion of care may be found in other locales of the disability imagination. Freakish and fantastic, the sadomasochistic care and collaborative art of Sheree Rose and the late Bob Flanagan treads back across the boundary of abuse to the notion of "self-abuse" (a coy ecclesiastical term for masturbation, invoking Flanagan's particular attention to his penis as a source of affliction). But Rose and Flanagan's abuse is in fact a form of care, a means of controlling the pain Flanagan experienced as a result of cystic fibrosis. Their *Visiting Hours* installation is remembered here in Karen Alkalay-Gut's awe-inspired and apologetically "banal" response, "Ode to Bob Flanagan."

Cynthia Margaret Gere's painting of embryos asphyxiating in bottles is an illustrative portrait from her essay, cowritten with Anne Ruggles Gere, on fetal alcohol syndrome, but it also suggests at its surface the current controversy around genetic engineering (babies in bottles) and "natural selection" (the abortion of fetuses with viable disabilities), which places disabled people in a second and undesirable category. Note that the Geres' attention to neglect has its political parallels: Elaine Makas and other academic activists in the disability rights movement point out that the cultural issue of "right to die" carries with it the fates of thousands of severely disabled children; their quality of life, consent, and right to live are determined by people who approximate appropriate care according to social norms rather than viability.[3] Medical care of the disabled is a major area of concern in our country at this time—most vehemently felt in the arrest of sixty-four members of ADAPT at the White House in November 1997 for illegally demonstrating over the stalling of MiCASA (Medical Community Attendant Service Act) in the House of Representatives. Still, Cynthia Gere's image impels a discussion of disabilities as a sequence of interpersonal and tribal effects, effects that cannot be treated medically, since they are about the adjustment of the world around the individual and not the disabled person himself or herself. An intriguing diagnosis, this failure to "cure" disabilities points us to other significant possibilities: first, the transformation of care from curing to sustenance; and, second, the recognition of disabilities that elude the attention of medical and other "experts" but that nonetheless affect a major dimension of everyday living.

"Living with Fetal Alcohol Syndrome / Fetal Alcohol Effect (FAS/FAE)" recreates a family lineage riddled with alternative possibilities and diverse expression; it seems conventional for a parent to speak of raising a learning-disabled child without expecting to be counterexamined, since parenting represents the central role for care among all conscious life. Here, however, mother and daughter offer alternating narratives, literary and visual; alternating cultures, white European American and Athabaskan Wolf Clan; alternating authorities, medical and Shaman healing. The Geres examine the relationship between giving care and establishing abilities. Who is giving care, who is careful? How does disability become represented in light of care, and does the meaning of care change when the recipient is disabled? While the Geres struggle for sober parity, Brooke Horvath's care for his child with Down's syndrome points out the poignant, asynchronous comedy of disabled children, ignorant tribes, and reading errors. The children's book *The Gingerbread Man,* a primer for literacy and for the connection between parent and child, provides the locus for Horvath's poetic contemplation. His daughter's mental disability causes schools, neighbors, even himself, to pursue his child in another "cookie-against-the-world" narrative; and we do, too, for this subject of fiction and life gingerly eludes social and learning norms with her choruses of "hello, hello, hello" to nervous passersby, inviting all readers into her elusive world. So who is the Gingerbread Man, the daughter or the poet?

We are left with a dual investigation: first, the role of art in constructing notions of disability; and, second, the role of disability as it constructs art. This collection offers points of contact in disability studies from within and without, by dovetailing art and disability in terms of the social relations each enables within the cultural imagination of Western culture. This volume represents the margins of disability as it is understood in its current identity politics (marked or "out" among disability circles in academic and artistic communities and made official by ADA eligibility, e.g.). Simultaneously, we have sought out studies of art that are cutting edge not so much in that they are avant-garde but, rather, that they are *sans garde,* without guard, art without clear defenders, owners, or even regard for that matter. In that sense we focus here on some of the stereotypical faces of disability—figures such as the victim, the freak, the patient, the client, and so forth—but then move beyond these types to the less visible and less symbolic exponents of disability: the independent disabled person, the disabled scholar, the disabled artist, the activist, people with learning disabilities, friends and family, the mentally and psychiatrically ill, lovers, people with eating disorders, the terminally ill, health professionals, the chronically fatigued, people with congenital differences, teachers, women with premenstrual syndrome, epileptics, and many more. We seek the experience of both disability and art as it involves daily living, production, creativity, and dedication—death, obstacle, destruction, and abuse. It is the familiar story of artists as they explore the unfamiliar. It is the familiar story of disability as it makes the familiar less so.

Rosemarie Garland Thomson and Victoria Ann Lewis are familiar practitioners within the field (and the story) of disability studies. In this volume each sets out (to borrow a phrase from Thomson) to "excavate the meaning of embodied differences" and the understanding of disabled and nondisabled body norms. In Thomson's explication of two central configurations of bodies within the cultural imagination of Western culture, the beauty and the freak, she explores narrative and ritual as the sources of theatrical dynamics related to the freak show and beauty pageant. Her scenario of acts and agencies permits an analysis of who watches, who performs, and what notions are reinforced through the "visual grammar" of exhibitions that generate a "hyperlegible . . . primary ideological language." These critiques represent art as ideative, or formulated within institutions, alongside art that, early in the game, poses problems and questions about the extent to which disability serves as an originary of culture.

Victoria Ann Lewis, whose seminal play *P*H*reaks* (1992–94) provides a historical synthesis of disability's place in the cultural imaginary, turns to the practicalities of her profession—she is a dramaturge and artistic director of the Mark Taper Forum OTHER VOICES project in Los Angeles. If, as her title suggests, there is a dramaturgy of disability, then disability must retain some original theater, one that contends with history and its stigma. From the annals of dramas-cum-screenplays—*Sunrise at Campbello, The Elephant Man,* and *Whose Life Is It Anyway?*—to recent work by Susan Nussbaum, Michael Ervin, Cheryl Marie Wade, John Belluso, and Brad Rothbart, Lewis fixes the dramaturgy of disability at a point intermediate to actor and audience.

Does art possess the potential to represent disability in ways that avow the term's unique and transforming effects in our civilization? Art, of course, is necessarily diverse and diverting, a cousin to both craft and cunning. Across the dimensional spectrum of high and low, presentation and representation, aestheticism and notoriety, "art" can be a helper to people with disabilities (wherefore art and music therapy), a servant to elite institutions and community framework, enablers of system stability or ideological revolution. Art can be personified as a helper, servant, master, and more. As several of our authors explore—for example, Karen Alkalay-Gut in her ode to Bob Flanagan—art aids civilization in its quest for perfection. In doing so, art paradoxically assumes both the aspect of the caregiver, and, speaking to the potential of disability studies for generating original perspectives of the world, the image and experience of disability. In a well-known essay on bodies, language, and caregiving titled "Plunging In," Nancy Mairs invites readers into a world fashioned in her image, shrunken to four feet eight, disabled by multiple sclerosis: "I ask you to read . . . not to be uplifted, but to be lowered and steadied into what may be unfamiliar, but is not inhospitable, space. Sink down beside me, take my hand, and together we'll watch the waists of the world drift past."[4] With artful collection, we offer our readers no certain body of disability, no standard height or privileged nondisabled body part with which to measure one's place in the disabled or nondisabled world. This text and its images offer something more valuable: the plausible composition of a disability imagination and the invitation to read the world afresh from the broadest spectrum of artistic life.

As an offering in the University of Michigan Press series Corporealities: Discourses of Disability, this book affirms the series' interest in the subject of the body as a source of rich interpretation and meaning. Thinking through disabled bodies and nondisabled bodies as "models" for such interpretation may lead to footfalls both similar and different to those that have run the path toward sex and gender. The writers and artists represented in this volume talk about bodies, yet they question rather than institute the body as the central figuration of humanity. Likewise, the status of disability and disability studies as territories (or as *a* discourse) is also questionable. *Territory* is a pure metaphor, something that cannot adequately express the richness of disability culture, since this culture coalesces with the greater one. Elspeth Morrison and Vic Finkelstein, working within the disability art movement in Britain, use the term *cultural intervention* to indicate disability's role in the revision of culture as a whole: "Helping disabled people to ensure an integrated role for disability arts and culture in the nation's repertoire of cultural life," they suggest, "can provide an opportunity to challenge narrow thinking, elitism and dependency on others."[5] The fact of disability in our culture is that there seem to be territories; for some, there is a war going on to reclaim America. As ADAPT blocks the steps of the Capitol with bodies and chairs or fights in the stead of those who lie in nursing homes, we are reminded that this territory was political before it became intellectual or aesthetic. The inspiration for academic vigilance and visibility, ADAPT has successfully transformed the representations of disabled people into a successful lobby; in the fall of 1997 Newt Gingrich introduced to the House the Medicaid Community Attendant Services Act, H.R. 2020, or MiCASA, which would legislate the right for disabled people to select the most appropriate care rather than accept assignment to nursing homes. Nursing homes, universities, and art centers make strange bedfellows in the grounding of a discipline, yet the politics of care and the assertion of identity seen in the works included here tell us that the claims of disability in our culture range far and wide and still cohere.

NOTES

1. Leonard Kriegel, "Falling into Life," in *Staring Back: The Disability Experience from the Inside Out,* ed. Kenny Fries (New York: Plume Books, 1997), 49.

2. Christopher Reeve's power to enact change did not disappear with the superhero that rights all wrongs nor with the appearance of a wife or parent at his side. The actor-director recently endorsed an H.R. 2020 bill on attendant care, prompting political disability lobbies to report that "Superman endorses MiCASA."

3. Elaine Makas, *End Results and Starting Points: Expanding the Field of Disability Studies* (Portland: Society of Disability Studies and The Edmund S. Muskie Institute, 1995), 21.

4. Nancy Mairs, *Waist High in the World: A Life among the Nondisabled* (Boston: Beacon Press, 1996), 18.

5. Elspeth Morrison and Vic Finkelstein, "Broken Arts and Cultural Repair: The Role of Culture in the Empowerment of Disabled People," in *Disabling Barriers, Enabling Environments,* ed. John Swain, Vic Finkelstein, Sally French, and Mike Oliver (London: Sage Publications /Open University, 1993). Reprinted on *Framed: Interrogating Disability in the Media,* ed. Ann Pointon and Chris Davies (London: British Film Institute, 1997), 165.

TOBIN SIEBERS

MY WITHERED LIMB

I am told that most people require an act of imagination to tell their right side from their left. My wife Jill, on whom I rely in matters of the imagination, transports herself to another time and another place and another body. She imagines herself a young girl again returned to her first school where they lined up the children with their left side to the curved wooden wall of the gymnasium and their right side to the open court. My daughter has been tutored by experts, like so many children today. The left hand, she tells me, is the one that makes true the letter L with index finger and thumb. Hold a hand aloft and know yourself.

I require neither trick of experts nor transport of imagination to tell my right from my left. My withered limb is my compass. It points right infallibly, although I fear sometimes that the meaning of rightness is hobbled by it. I think of it as my chicken-bone leg because it has grown longer over time but not thicker and looks like a leftover on a plate. It is meatless, thinner at points than the wrist of my right hand, and deformed by years of exertion. The neat little cap that most people know as their ankle begins where it should on the inside of my foot but exits where it shouldn't on the outside at the Achilles tendon. To the untutored eye, it looks as if I have no ankle bone at all. My toes are curled under, some beneath the others, the toenails thin and milky white, like a newborn's, always with rotting skin. I know which side is my right because this is what God has attached to me.

Poliomyelitis struck during my second year of life. It struck down a lot of small children and adults that year, the same year Dr. Jonas Salk perfected his vaccination, and wide-scale immunization began. The vaccination didn't get to me in time, but I have a small consolation. I am the luckiest in my acquaintance—

lungs intact, no arms affected, one leg not two—except for everyone in my acquaintance who was not struck down. 1955 knew one of the hottest summers on record, and heat breeds polio. I was in the kitchen with my mother. Chocolate chip cookies were sizzling on a flat pan in the oven, the linoleum floor was cool, and I could not get up off of it. The doctor said I was only pretending. My mother said I wasn't that kind of child. Later he ate his words and made the diagnosis. They took me to the hospital and put me in quarantine. I screamed at the slammed door all night long, "Daddy! Daddy! I want to go home!" On the other side, my father listened to my muffled cries, giving him his first taste of impotent rage. Me, too. Speculation was that I had caught it at a backyard cookout where fish guts were too much in evidence. My mother also remembered finding me playing jacks in the dirt on the corner of Eden and Whitney. She should have known better, she felt. Or maybe she should have breastfed me. That's what the doctor said.

This last bit of history I report by hearsay. The rest of what I will tell you I know because I remember it. I will try not to wallow in self-pity, fool you with false machismo, or get too philosophical—all temptations when you are exhibiting your own wounds—but I will likely succumb to all three. This is because what I have to tell you is understandable only in these terms. There are no other models of explanation, at least not in the America I know. To be crippled in America is not the American way. In a country where image is everything, it is hard to find an example for growing up crippled and hardly worth it when you do. The icon of the cripple is paralytic, a double-edged sword, but we desire role models all the same. They tried to make one of FDR last year, setting him in stone upon his wheelchair, condemning him to a double immobility. A wheelchair made of stone is an interesting object for any paralyzed person to contemplate. My example was Chester, the crippled sidekick of Marshall Dillon in *Gunsmoke.* Not often but often enough, throughout grade school, "Chester" was my nickname. Boys from strange neighborhoods who made incursions into ours would mock me across an open field or yard with exaggerated stumbles while yelling in their best Western accent, "Mr. Dillon! Mr. Dillon!" That should have made me the Marshall, but my own hobbled gait proved that I was more the sidekick than they.

I was a role model myself for a short time. Never the exalted poster child for the March of Dimes, I was nevertheless the poster child of choice for the newsletter at my father's work-place. I don't know what effect this had on other polio victims. I still have a picture of myself in physical therapy with Dr. Veracka, whom I remember most for the electrical tickles he gave me and his surprising bow ties. I am sporting my favorite T-shirt of the era, featuring a drawing of Pinky Lee, another bumbling side-kick of a Western hero, this time of Roy Rogers, who is exclaim-ing, "Yoo-Hoo! It's me, Pinky Lee!" In my own caption, I am in-forming Dr. Veracka, "That tickles!" When he wasn't using electrodes on me, he would run a closed ball-point pen against the bottom of my foot, the underside of my knee, and other ten-der spots. I liked Dr. Veracka and much preferred this trick to the technique of other doctors who used a safety pin to jab me and still do to this day.

When I was twelve I made the headlines again. It was my last time as an exemplum for the lame. I was on the frozen Fox River with my brother and friends. We were making holes in the ice. The preferred method was to find a very large rock, run out onto the ice, and dash it against the surface. My brother bragged that he was going to make the biggest hole in the ice. But his rock was too big to handle, and he threw it down at his own feet. The rock broke through the ice with a splash, and so did he. While the other boys gawked, I ran over to help him out of the fast and freezing waters. He was already on his way to safety and only required my hand on his wet mitten. Nevertheless, the headline, "Kaukauna Boy Pulls Brother from Fox River," fed to the newspaper by the mother of a cowardly witness, made me the hero, although the article added a cautionary note in its final sentence about the limits of hobbled heroism: "Tobin has polio of the right leg and fortunately was relatively close to his brother when the accident occurred." To this day, I remind my brother when he gets testy that I saved his life. "But only because you were relatively close," he retorts.

I wonder whether my fellow handicappers identified at the time with my brush with fame, whether they found some conso-lation in my appearance on a small world stage. Perhaps they viewed it with the same irony that I do now. Probably not, since irony requires a certain knowledge of the self, and those search-ing for images of self lack this knowledge or they wouldn't be looking so hard.

The human eye is fascinated by the powerful lines of the hero. We love in America what is beautiful and perfect and healthy. We hate the rest and tolerate it only with unease. But the human eye is fascinated as well by the broken curves of the cripple. The latter is actually the more natural impulse. The unfit die, Darwin found, when they are made visible to the predator. The cruel eye of the lioness on the hot savannah targets the zebra whose wobbling gait breaks the dizzying pattern of black and white, and he falls prey to her hunger and ferocity, scarlet splattered on his stripes at the feasting. Human beings have no hunger for their own kind, lame or not, but their eyes are no less cruel, even when they are trying to be kind. An armless man enters the elevator where I am standing. It is winter, but he is wearing a sleeveless T-shirt, his blunt, fleshy fins protruding to either side. I understand immediately that he stands atop artificial limbs because he is covered in sweat and breathing hard. The exertion of movement is so strenuous for him, so beyond the human body and its capacity to cool itself down, that he requires no protection against the cold and must pray at times for the frost to form. I stare at him transfixed and then look down at the floor quickly when he meets my eyes, like everyone else in the elevator. The key is the "like everyone else." I have been rendered instantly more normal by my friend's presence. We are never more normal than when we catch sight of a cripple. This applies to the fit and unfit alike.

A week later I am walking into the building, jammed with people, where I have my office. Walking just ahead of me is another cripple, limping exactly with my trademark rhythm, rocking from side to side, like a metronome. Now we are two. Tick tock, tick tock. Into the door we go. Tick tock, tick tock. Down the hall one after the other in a row. Tick tock, tick tock. One cripple is invisible compared to two cripples. Two cripples walking in a line are a comedy act. We are today's show. He doesn't know I am behind him, but he knows something is wrong. The people crowding past him and streaming toward me have that strange expression on their face, an expression that he and I know only too well, but what has caused such an epidemic today, he wonders? Finally, he looks over his shoulder, sees me, and figures it out. "Take a hike," his look tells me. The same message he reads on my face. I have never had another cripple seek me out for company in a crowded room, the way women flock to women,

men to men, children to children, and human stripe to human stripe, whether black, white, yellow, or red. We are strangers to each other.

The solitude of the disabled is crushing. We are barred from gathering among ourselves by the laws of human physics, which declare that gravity exerts five times its influence where two cripples stand in one place, ten times its influence where four of us gather. All objects slump close to the horizon and threaten to crash to the earth where the burden of weight finds its final rest. Gravity is shifting, but there is no danger of earthquakes. No faults will crack and churn the earth. A new landscape is in the process of being formed, and it has its own vastness and glory, like the beauty of the western states of America where the land is low and the sky has more air to fill with light. And yet the upright and the healthy fear the leveling of the horizon. They are afraid they will be brought low themselves and swallowed by the dirt. They forbid our gathering with looks and ridicule; we accept their judgment and drive ourselves into seclusion. A motorized wheelchair, its withered inhabitant inclining forward in determination of movement, inches snail-like along the wall of a hallway crowded with people. They are gesturing and telling stories, laughing and arguing in a celebration of everything human, but not one of them will notice, let alone speak to, the boy in the wheelchair who waits with virtuoso patience for the human sea to part for him. His inertia immerses him day in and day out in the colors and details of other human lives, but he is always alone.

People see the crippled other as other than themselves no matter who they are and experience irony at this fact only after repeated bouts of self-consciousness. The more immediate response is revulsion that can lead in a fraction of a second to real violence. Every disabled person has been the victim of it at one time or another. We live in an age some have called the Age of the Victim, where we all want to be identified with the long suffering, as long as we aren't really in pain, so let's be clear for a moment about what history teaches us about the disabled. No human group has ever been so subject to violence, none so marginalized. In ancient Greece we were left to die on the cold mountain hillsides, in Africa we were food for beasts, in Europe dropped down a well. People forget the Nazis perfected their death machine on the disabled before they moved on to the

Gypsies and Jews. Visit an orphanage in any civilized country today, and see who is abandoned there: the deformed, the maimed, the diseased, the mentally impaired.

A white man will lynch a black man to favor his own color. A man will rape a woman for the sport of other men. Nations will destroy other nations for no reason other than self-love. It is only a matter of turning our kind against their kind. The disabled fall out of the orbit of mundane prejudice because everyone agrees about their contemptibility: white men beat up white cripples, women of all kinds and colors desert their own children if maimed, the only nation of the disabled is the nation of the abandoned and the dead. History is not on our side. Neither is God. He will not pluck a rib from me and set it free as womanly flesh.

So much for the truth. But since this truth comes with heavy doses of self-pity, I say, "Down with the truth." Let no one know or think about it. Pity is more loathsome to the cripple than anything else. We have spent all of our lives trying to be normal, trying to pass the test, trying to run with the pack, to be liked and not pitied. To show self-pity is to add defect to defect, and more defect we do not want. That is why you do not see much of it. No special favors is the rule of the day. Gym class was the only time as a boy when I could remove my brace. They said my street shoes would ruin the gym floor, so with delight I donned tennis shoes like the other children. The morning exercise was to leap over a jump rope, time after time, as it was raised higher and higher. No problem at the lower levels. But the higher levels presented a quandary. If I pushed off with my dead leg and led with my good, I would fall on my face in front of everyone. If I pushed off with my good leg, I would land with full force on my bad leg and hurt myself. Of course, I could jump with both feet at the same time, but that would not be leaping, and leaping I wanted to be. So I leapt and cracked my bad ankle against the floor. Later in the office, where the call to my mother was being made, the gym teacher explained to the principal, "They want so to be like the other children and don't like to be left out."

And so for years I went on forced marches, stumbling for miles and miles. When my father asked if I wanted the family car, I said my brother could have it. I took the stairs and shunned elevators. I cut my own lawn, hung my own storm windows, dangled on ladders, and stood on the roof. I was the first to give up my seat on buses and the subway. I still walk ten feet ahead of my own family when we are en route anywhere, leading the way and setting the pace.

But I have been fooling myself. It has all been an elaborate sight gag staged for my own ego. And I am beginning to pay the price for it. Years of overexertion and bravado have taken their toll on my muscles and joints. I first noticed it when I had small children. Children need to be carried. I could once carry a suit-case for a mile, if I had to, through sheer determination. But I could not carry a two-year old for three blocks, no matter how hard I tried, because I need my arms for balance and the added weight turns my legs to stone. I especially could not carry children up staircases, this being one thing they most need you to do. I began to notice that other people were picking up my children and carrying them around. Then I found myself begging out of evening walks with the family. Ladders became fearsome objects. Two-story house tours at dinner parties are no longer fun. My backyard is currently full of unraked leaves. My daughter raked the front lawn two weeks ago. The hoax is over.

I believe I have been in denial for forty years and even now invent little lies to explain my "new" condition to myself. I know how it happened to me, I think. It was because my lucky shoes wore out. I had them for ten years, and they made me unstoppable, but the minute I threw them away, my legs gave way. Or, perhaps, it was those round silver panels embossed with the blue wheelchair that you now see next to so many doors. I started to get lazy, and I pushed them whenever I could. They open the door automatically for you, and you walk through like a king. But they also do something else. They cut the legs out from under you. I pushed that panel when I didn't have to, and I didn't realize I was placing an order for my own wheelchair.

It looks like I am going to be needing some help with my life. The leaves keep falling from the trees, and the grass is growing by the minute. There are things upstairs that I need when I am downstairs, and vice versa. How to go about asking for help with dignity? How to accept charity when it is offered? Twenty-five years ago I witnessed one of the most bizarre lessons in charity I have ever seen. I was walking in the street. It was a sunny January day but bitterly cold. A blind man was standing with his cane on a busy corner, hoping to make a safe crossing. He was hatless, had short-cropped hair, and his large ears were turning from blue to bloodless white. I walked over to him and asked if he needed help crossing the street. "No!" he said bluntly. So I crossed and left him behind. But I was feeling a little worried about him, so I looked back over my shoulder to assure myself. Someone else was helping him cross the street. I paused to watch them make the crossing. His savior left him and pursued her own course. Then I saw the blind man position himself to cross back to his previous location. People came up to him and offered assistance. He refused them. Then he accepted someone and crossed to the other corner, where within moments he repositioned himself to make the crossing again. I watched him replay this little drama until my own endurance failed against the cold. He had made a ritual out of charity. Those who thought he was powerless and stopped to offer their help would discover who had the last word about power. I now understand this man, but I don't want to become him.

I am reading the *Handbook on the Late Effects of Poliomyelitis for Physicians and Survivors*. Perhaps it will teach me something about my current condition. It is full of valuable facts about polio survivors, and I am one of them. *Physics*: The muscles of polio survivors cannot meet daily demands, so they are regularly assisted by some "substitutive posturing." Consequently, polio survivors work abnormally hard (2.5 times as hard as normal) to accomplish the same activity: walking, sports, etc. The added strain may result in "overuse damage." Chronic strain on joints being used in abnormal ways often leads to early degenerative changes. Common musculoskeletal problems include osteoarthritis of the spine and of peripheral joints, scoliosis, bursitis, tendonitis, osteoporosis, myofascial pain syndromes, foot and toe deformities, carpal tunnel syndrome, and chronic postural strain to back and neck muscles producing chronic pain. *Biology*: In polio survivors, who already have reduced cell populations, age-related loss of cells may produce enough weakness to interfere with normal activities such as walking. Muscles weakened by polio cannot in general be strengthened by an exercise program, which may only enhance "cell death" and create "a cycle of ever-increasing weakness." *Psychology*: Polio survivors often have a low tolerance for gadgetry. And yet a person who has walked normally may begin to need a cane, a person who has used braces and crutches may need to use a wheelchair, a manual wheelchair user may need to change to a motorized wheelchair, and a power chair user may need "further adaptive equipment." These changes require an open mind. When a person's "level of functional independence" is changed, depression and sadness are normal. *Medical Ethics*: Many polio survivors have been labeled "hypochondriac" or "neurotic," have been given inappropriate prescriptions, or have been sent off for seemingly endless, expensive referrals. A frequent complaint of polio survivors is that the doctors do not appear to listen to them. *Conclusion*: It is imperative that polio survivors educate themselves about their condition and learn to conserve energy.

I am back in physical therapy again after forty years of freedom. My therapist is named Maryanne. She is teaching me low-impact exercises, like back extensions, hip abductions, and hip extensions, and trying to talk me into wading in a swimming pool for ten minutes every day. I like her almost as much as Dr. Veracka, even though she doesn't wear bow ties, because she is coy and ferociously honest at the same time. When I arrive for my appointment, she meets me at the door, hiding something behind her back and smiling like a lover. It is a cane. I am hesitant to try it, so she tells me a story about her grandfather. He refused to wear a hearing aid because he was afraid it would make him look too old. "But Grandpa," the punch line goes, "you're eighty and you have no hair." The moral of the story is easily applied to me: "You're used to the way you look when you walk and probably think a cane will make you look funny. But most people already think you look funny." I take the cane from her, even though I don't want to touch it. As far as I'm concerned, this staff has already turned into a serpent. She moves it gently from my right to my left hand, which is surprising. I have always dreaded using a cane because I thought I wouldn't be able to keep my right hand free. I realize that I know nothing about the physics of impaired walking, although I've been doing it for some time. Maryanne explains how the cane works. I make my way awkwardly around the room, trying to get the feel of the cane and synchronizing it with the steps of my right foot. She tells me to speed up, and I find I can walk as fast as I want. My frame no longer crumples at the waist with each step. My back is no longer in pain—an odd sensation since I had not realized that I was previously in pain. The pain of forty years from a wound I was pretending not to have quiets to a whisper in my body.

The self is a scar, Freud said. Everyone is a different wound healed over. But the wounds of the disabled often refuse to heal. They are not like cuts or bruises or broken bones. They are disabled wounds—that is what makes them so hard to accept by the firm and infirm alike—but they define who we are, nevertheless. My withered limb is who I am. It is right for me. This is no idle pun but flesh of my being. The meaning of rightness would not be the same for me if God had not taken my right leg from me. My leg is right because it is everything I am and everything I could not be.

I am not like any of you, and I don't want to be like any of them. I am who I am.

I am my withered limb.

JOSEPH GRIGELY

POSTCARDS TO SOPHIE CALLE

Author's Note: The "Postcards to Sophie Calle" were written in the spring of 1991, as a response to Sophie Calle's exhibition, *Les Aveugles*, at Luhring Augustine Gallery in New York. A selection of 16 of the "Postcards" was published in English and German in the Swiss art quarterly, *Parkett* (No. 36, 1993, pp. 88-101). For the present publication I have collected together all 32 of the original "Postcards."

Dear Sophie,

I am writing to you about your New York show at Luhring Augustine in the spring of 1991, particularly one installation: *Les Aveugles*. My curiosity—or is it my concern?—is a reflection of anomalies and ambiguities: New York with its unforgiving inaccessibility is not a city of patience, nor is Luhring Augustine an artspace where one expects the voice of an oppressed minority; and you, Sophie Calle, a professed voyeur of private lives, what is this installation you present to us?

On a small pedestal in the center of the room is a lectern on which is placed the conceptual locus of *Les Aveugles*: "*I met people who were born blind. Who had never seen. I asked them what their image of beauty was.*"

Around the room framed texts record the responses of these people: brief, printed declarations of beauty. I—like others around me—am easily taken in by these voices and their resonance:

> What pleases me aesthetically is a man's body, strong and muscular.

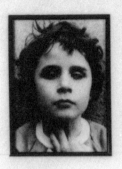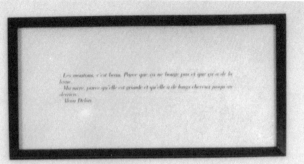

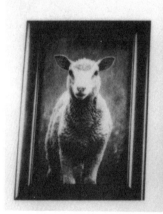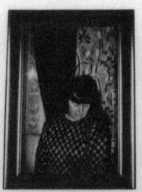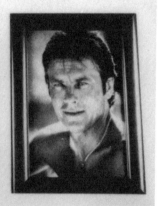

An artwork from Sophie Calle's exhibit, *Les Aveugles*. In response to the question, what beauty is, this girl responds in the printed text:

> "Sheep, that's beautiful. Because they don't move and because they have wool."

> "My mother is beautiful too, because she's tall and her hair goes down to her bottom."

> "Alain Delon."

From *Sophie Calle: A Survey,* curated by Deborah Irmas, Fred Hoffman Gallery, Santa Monica, California

Hair is magnificent. Especially African hair. I curl up in women's long hair. I pretend I'm a cat and meow.

In the Rodin Museum, there is a naked woman with very erotic breasts and a terrific ass. She is sweet, she is beautiful.

I am—how shall I say it?—entranced. No other word will do.

Yours,

Joseph

Dear Sophie,

My entrancement is mitigated by something troubling about these words, and what is troubling is that they are, shall we say, *forthright*. They do not apologize for the fact that it is the body, the engendered body particularly, that must be touched to be seen. This is the tactile gaze of the blind. It is a gaze unconditioned by whatever feminism and sexual politics have taught us about touching. The terms and conditions by which this tactile gaze exists thus cannot be judged by our own standard, where the actions of the blind become rendered—I use that word advisedly—into *our* vocabulary of tactile violence. This touching is not about feeling, not about touching even, but about seeing. Touching itself is elided; it is a semantic projection of our own physiology, not that of the blind. If everyone in the world were blind, perhaps touching would be called seeing.

Am I being too romantic? Quite possibly. But inasmuch as the Deaf do not see sign language as a pretty way of communicating—it's language, language pure and simple—I think the same can be said about this tactile gaze: it's about seeing, not about touching. This is the inevitable effect of an imposed transmodality: it reconfigures our physiological conventions and the language with which we describe those conventions. This room and the voices of the people within it require much patience, Sophie. I need to slow down here, we all need to slow down and begin to try to understand what is behind this tactile gaze—we need to rediscover the act of seeing, and should we freeze up at the sight—*our* sight—of this seeing-as-touching, it is our preconceptions that freeze us and our unwillingness—not inability, but unwillingness—to see what we are seeing.

And what are we seeing, Sophie?

Yours,

Joseph

Dear Sophie,

Beguiled now, I am almost afraid to face the photographs that supplement these texts, almost afraid to go past the honest audacity of this language to that which lies beyond: images that presume to be of the objects, people, places, and passions described. But here they are: the Rodin, her erotic breasts and terrific ass flattened by ektachrome into two dimensions; a woman's head covered with blond hair; a man's body tangled in sheets. Yet, the most troubling part remains: your photographs of the faces of these blind people: their signatures. I am arrested by the fact that these images do not, because of their visual modality, return themselves to the blind. *Since your face is not available to me, why should my face be available to you?* An echo from somewhere, but I cannot pin it down. Something seems wrong to me: I am able to gaze, look, stare into the faces, into the eyes, of faces and eyes that cannot stare back. "Subjects," they are called. I feel I am in the presence of a social experiment. I feel I am being watched, feel as if I am a part of this experiment. Alone and not alone, I am uncomfortable.

Yours,

Joseph

Dear Sophie,

I hate myself here, yet I am taken in, seduced, drawn closer to this cultural keyhole. I struggle with my ambivalences—don't we all, don't you?—struggle with these images: hypostatization, the inscribed voice, and Sophie Calle's photographic interpretation of that voice. I look closer at the voices, try to listen, try to expunge the images that intervene—the faces, the photographs, the presence of Sophie Calle. It isn't easy. The photographs of the voices, your photographs, your interpretations, are resolutely hermeneutic: they crowd around me, crowd around the texts, impose themselves, and in the end reveal not so much the voices of the blind as the voice of Sophie Calle. I turn from the keyhole; I feel guilty, angry. Pushing away, I push myself closer.

Yours,

Joseph

Dear Sophie,

One thing becoming clear just now is that recent cultural representations of the disabled are often, it seems, mediated by those who are from outside the experience: Nicholas Nixon's photographs of blind children, Frederick Wiseman's documentary films on schools for the Deaf and the blind, and Nancy Burson's photographs of children with cranio-facial disorders. All of these works have, I must admit, brilliant, sensitive, and (in)sightful moments, but they simultaneously evince a certain awkwardness in the fact that they remain "documentary" works. They are, that is, representations that are at best interpretations, like your own photographs. Looking at this art people remain on the outside looking in, looking in through the camera's eye, looking in through the double turn of culture and aesthetics—looking in, that is, at the inextricable tangle of truth and fiction, at a tangle that will never, can never, untangle itself. Nor, I suppose, can we.

Yours,

Joseph

Dear Sophie,

I'm stepping back now, stepping outside of this room, stepping into the register of contemporary critical discourse and thoughts about how issues concerning the disabled fit into paradigms of this discourse. Perhaps you are aware that one acknowledgment of postcolonial criticism is how our predecessors engaged in cultural voyeurism and aesthetic appropriation. Both in art and literature modernism arguably owes much of its existence to the confluence of "primitive" aesthetics and discourse. By reifying aspects of the colonized other into a western whitemale ethos, our cultural practices evolved as a mode of "refined" (and hence permissible, even desirable) barbarism. Perhaps unconsciously, this barbarism remains within us, remains—dare I say it?—within your work: the other is not a colonized other living elsewhere, but a native other, a physiological other living in our midst. Why have you transcribed the voices of the blind into a medium to which they do not have access? What difference is there between gazing at the eyes of the blind or the labia of the Hottentot Venus? It is a discomfiting analogy, and I realize some people will not like it. They will be angry. Perhaps then they will begin to understand the anger of the disabled—how the gaze that acts under the guise of curiosity, like colonialist curiosity, is actually a gaze of violence. We are at a stage in cultural history where our conceptions of "otherness," to be truly other, must move beyond representations of the canonized Other. The colonized no longer necessarily live abroad; they live next door to us, and within our own homes.

Yours,

Joseph

Dear Sophie,

Despite my initial resistance to your work, I sense that there is something uniquely engaging about *Les Aveugles*. Part of my ambivalence is in realizing that what strikes me in a negative way is striking others quite differently. Is this because I am disabled and others are not? Is this because I see, as others perhaps do not, a convoluted relationship between the studied history of colonization and the (largely) unstudied history of the disabled? Is this because I see emerging from these texts the horror of domestic colonization? "Colonization" is of course a strong word, because it suggests subjection through the use of physical force.

But frightful too—perhaps more frightful when one realizes how subtle and psychologically tortuous it is—is the use of language as a colonizing agent. The oppression of native languages and attempts to control the genesis of a language by other means (what is most often termed "language planning") is an undeniable aspect of the history of many oppressed people. More difficult to acknowledge as oppression is when the language one social group uses to discuss another social group marks itself in negative terms: the identity is branded—"marked"—by language. Metaphor, particularly, is a form of latent violence that becomes manifest in the use of blindness and deafness as pejorative metaphors to imply ignorance, witlessness, and stupidity.

The phenomenon is ingrained, a reflection of how easily the disabled are stereotyped, and, in its ongoing pervasiveness, a reflection of how the changes related to racism and sexism in language have not yet been felt by the disabled. The English language has yet to respond to the vast semantic space between not being able to see and not being willing to see, between being unable to hear and being unwilling to hear. This, for example, is Elaine Showalter, writing in *Raritan* (Fall 1983):

> We can hardly fail to welcome male feminist criticism when we have so long lamented the blindness, the deafness, and indifference of the male critical establishment toward our work.

This is Kwame Anthony Appiah, writing in *Critical Inquiry* (Winter 1991):

> All aspects of contemporary African cultural life—including music and some sculpture and painting, even some writings with which the West is largely not familiar—have been influenced, often powerfully, by the transition of African societies *through* colonialism, but they are not all in the relevant sense *post*colonial. For the *post-* in postcolonial, like the *post-* in postmodernism, is the *post-* of the space-clearing gesture I characterized earlier, and many areas of contemporary African cultural life—what has come to be theorized as popular culture, in particular—are not in this way concerned with transcending, with going beyond, coloniality. Indeed, it might be said to be a mark of popular culture that its borrowings from international cultural forms are remarkably insensitive to, not so much dismissive of as blind to, the issue of neocolonialism or "cultural imperialism."

And this—it's a long quotation but needs a full citation—is from an artists' statement by Houston Conwill, Joseph De Pace, and Estella Conwill Majozo that accompanied their 1992 installation at the Brooklyn Museum:

> We create maps of language that present cultural pilgrim-ages and metaphorical journeys of transformation that can be experienced as rites of passage through life and death to re-birth and resurrection, fostering greater cultural awareness and understanding. They are composed of collaged and edited quotations from world music including spirituals, blues, gospel, soul, jazz, funk, samba, merengue, reggae, rap music, and freedom songs in dialect, and critical voicings from speeches of heroic models of African-American culture. Their prophetic and humanistic words reflect the values and aspira-tions of the culture—hope, wisdom, temperance, justice, and love—and function as both a critique and a healing, address-ing issues of world peace, social justice, human rights, civil rights, rights of the physically challenged, freedom, equality, democracy, history, memory, cultural identity, loss, cultural di-versity, multicultural education, pro-choice, public support for the arts, ecology, and caring. They also address the universal enemies of war, hatred, racism, oppression, classism, violence, bigotry, censorship, sickness, drug addiction, sexism, ageism, apartheid, homelessness, AIDS, greed, imperialism, colonial-ism, militarism, historical and cultural amnesia, cross-cultural blindness, and fear of the Other.

Cross-cultural blindness? It is almost ironic, Sophie, that the peo-ple who continue to use these pejorative metaphors are also the people who have done the most to open our cultural conscious-ness to the diversity of the human condition. *Almost* ironic; what else, Sophie, can it mean?

Yours,

Joseph

Dear Sophie,

I have a hypothesis about the English language and how our sensitivity toward human differences is aligned with certain linguistic factors: terms like "racism" and "sexism" work successfully in English because they use a monosyllable in an easily engaged disyllabic form, and this adds to their ubiquitous presence in everyday discourse. Hence, it is easy to see how such terms and their concomitant ideologies are more readily assimilated by the American population: "race" and "sex" are quick draws. "Disabled"—already an inadequate term—is trisyllabic, burdened with awkwardness. "Differently abled"; "physically challenged"; "handicapped": none of these terms works, nor have we a term to describe conscious and unconscious oppression of the disabled ("paternalism" comes close, but as a metaphor it does its own share of unjust damage). Defeated by the aporia of language and the strictures of etymology we crawl back into our present: we are we to ourselves alone. You remain you. The gulf widens.

Yours,

Joseph

Dear Sophie,

I have a little more to say about language today, about semantics particularly—that is, about meanings and connotations.

My concern just now is about why the disabled as a social group have made little progress in becoming a central part of our social consciousness. I mean, Sophie, when people talk about "multi-culturalism," they seem to mean everyone except the disabled—we're something else. *Something else.* I'm sure there are many reasons why this categorizing occurs—some are political, some demographic, some educational—but the most important reason, I think, is linguistic.

A large part of the problem is that the word "disabled" is not exclusively applied to humans or human culture. When we speak of "African-Americans" or "Asians," or adjectival variations ("African-American history," "Asian culture," and so on), we identify a human nexus from which consequent human activity originates. We are thus constantly reminded of the human center, that it is a people, even a diverse people, not an ideology, that is at the root of signification. But this is not so for the disabled: the word "disabled" does not automatically engage a human context because it is part of an independent matrix for that which is dysfunctional or otherwise adjudicated by prefixes: *dis*abled, *ab*normal, *mal*functional. On the New Jersey Turnpike between Delaware and New York are a great number of signs that, as social texts, reiterate this matrix: "Please park disabled cars behind cones"; "Please wait with disabled vehicles." What the matrix continually communicates is that a disabling condition is a deviant condition, one which subverts an illusory normalcy and needs assistance of some kind to restore ("rehabilitate") it to a more socially accepted condition.

This is important, because the matrix assures us that society will continue to see the disabled in the same way that it sees its automobiles: in need of new fan belts, patched tires, and overhauled engines. It is not a people at the center of being, but a dysfunction. And we cannot easily undo this matrix: we cannot say "Please park broken cars behind cones" because, though semantically honest, it does not have the psychological imperative that the word "disabled" conveys. Our world is a world made of metaphors: they make language, they make ideas, and they even make poetry, but they also unmake people.

Yours,

Joseph

Dear Sophie,

Every time I get a bit of space to relax, that echo keeps coming back to me: *Since your face is not available to me, why should my face be available to you?*—There is something about this utterance that is both searching and defiant, something about it that stops short of absolute resistance. Perhaps it is the curl of the question mark that dares us, hanging on to the final word, *you.*

Today it came back to me. The voice I mean; its origin. It's from John Hull's *Touching the Rock: An Experience of Blindness* (New York, 1990):

> Another aspect . . . is the horror of being faceless, of forgetting one's own appearance, of having no face. The face is the mirror image of the self.

Is this linked with the desire which I sometimes feel to strongly hide my face from others? I want to hold my chin and to cover my mouth with one hand, pressing my hand against my nose, as if I were wearing a mask. Is this a primitive desire to find some kind of equality? Since your face is not available to me, why should my face be available to you? Or does it spring from a sense that the face has been lost? Am I somehow mourning over the loss of the face? Am I trying to regain the assurance that I have got a face by feeling it with my own hands? I want to touch my very lips as I am speaking. Other people's voices come from nowhere. Does my own voice also come from nowhere?

I can't say more.

Yours,

Joseph

Dear Sophie,

Friday, March 22nd. I have returned to your show and purchased a catalogue. It is a catalogue from your 1989 exhibition at the Fred Hoffman Gallery in Santa Monica, but it is all that the gallery here has. In the introduction, Deborah Irmas—she curated your show there, yes?—writes:

> What is so compelling about this project is its didactic function. We measure our notions of beauty (which most of us seldom think about) against the simplistic but often heartfelt responses of the subjects.

I look again at the inscribed voices:

> Flowers bother me, I'm afraid to step on them.

> My mother stopped me from touching things. She would say: "Don't touch, it makes you look like a blind person."

> I don't need beauty, I don't need images in my brain.

> I've never come across absolute perfection.

> I believe what I want to believe.

. . . "simplistic"?

Yours,

Joseph

Dear Sophie,

The New Yorker has printed a brief description of your show in the gallery listings for April 8th. In part, it goes like this:

> Calle interviewed a number of people who were born blind, asking them to describe their images of beauty, then illustrating these definitions by taking pictures of the subjects and what they described. Some of these people look blind, some of them don't.

I stop at that last sentence, re-read it: *Some of these people look blind, some of them don't.* I am not sure what exactly this means, how it is intended to mean; yet it somehow means much in an unbearably unpredictable way. The very idea of looking blind, of bearing visible signs of identity, is somehow striking: one thinks of Paul Strand's photograph of a blind woman, a string with a signcard placed around her neck: "BLIND." Look at the xerox copy I've enclosed. To what extent should otherness be a visible attribute? Would *The New Yorker* say of Robert Mapplethorpe's photographs: "Some of these people look homosexual, some of them don't"?

I look into a mirror at myself, search for my deafness, yet fail to find it. For some reason we have been conditioned to presume difference to be a visual phenomenon, the body as the locus of race and gender. Perhaps I need a hearing aid, not a flesh-colored one but a red one: a signifier that leaves little room for discursiveness, a signifier that ceremoniously announces itself. But I know too that the moment I open my mouth my nasal sibilants will give me away; I know that the moment you speak to me behind my back you will think I am ignoring you. It is a scenario that is a cliché, yet a cliché that is at times unbearably real. Once, at the Metropolitan Museum of Art, while sitting on the floor as I spent time with David's *Marat*, a museum guard struck me on the shoulder and berated me for not getting up on my feet the first time he warned me.

Some of these people look blind, some of them don't.

Yours,

Joseph

Dear Sophie,

Can I tell you a story? It is not the sort of story that we describe as a tale with a moral, but a real story that is itself a moral.

One evening an acquaintance of mine, visiting New Orleans, went straight to the French Quarter for the sort of reasons people go to New Orleans: for the vibrations of jazz, the rhythms of blues, and the carnivalesque atmosphere that makes the French Quarter what it is. For her it was an inviting thing to do, and for a while at least it was inviting indeed. But then, early in the evening, something happened. A policeman had noticed her unsteady gait and stopped her to ask a few questions. She could not, however, understand him very well, nor did he understand her responses. He was a smart policeman and knew intoxication when he saw it.

She was arrested for public drunkenness. Her arrest record cites her "slurred speech," her "uncomprehending behavior," and her "erratic movement." She spent a very long night alone in jail trying to understand why she was arrested for being everything she was, everything she could possibly be: a young deaf woman with cerebral palsy.

Some of these people look blind, some of them don't.

Yours,

Joseph

Dear Sophie,

You might think that Joseph's story is a lie, a fiction. But when I first heard it—I—along with fourteen students who shared a

room with this woman—recognized at once not the verisimili-
tude of the story (for there is almost none), but its raw truth: for
us, all sixteen of us deaf, it was familiar, too familiar, a familiar
surrealism that makes our lives inexplicable and unbelievable to
everyone except ourselves.

And that is why, when we read books and see movies about the
lives of disabled people, we recognize that these are not real
lives, but lives filtered through the ideologies of able-bodied people, lives that are made believable so that they can be marketed
to a believing audience.

Like *Les Aveugles*.

Yours,

Joseph

Dear Sophie,

My last postcard was perhaps a bit strong. I'm sorry for that.
Truth is rarely polite.

You must be wondering: what is Joseph's agenda, what is the
agenda of this person who questions and vilifies Sophie Calle for
her aesthetics and her parsimonious gesture of magnanimity?

I will try to explain.

Part of the problem is (as I suggested in an earlier postcard)
related to representations of the disabled, and what are more
generally discussed as "authentic" and "inauthentic" representations of racial and sexual difference. These are really difficult
terms to qualify and they substantiate themselves only by virtue
of the fact that they provide the grounds for an ongoing cultural
debate, the tension by which culture necessarily sustains, perpetuates, and remakes itself. I may chastise you, Sophie, but I cannot correct you. In the realm of cultural exchanges everything
that is right for somebody is wrong for somebody else.

It is not an ideology I am sending you in these postcards; there
is no theoretical locus here, but only a theoretical tangle, a tangle of frayed perceptions about the disabled as a part of the network of human differences. How, Sophie, can we measure and
quantify something so abstract as difference? Why should we? We

are all tangled in each other: Joseph, Sophie, *Les Aveugles*. All of us different, all of us equal in our differences.

A contradiction, yes. There are many of them, and that is my purpose here: to peel back the contradictions of ideology, not to create an ideology that represses contradictions. I would not be honest to you or to myself if what I said did not also reflect the chaos of who and what we are.   .

Yours,

Joseph

Dear Sophie,

Among the reviews and observations of your earlier exhibition of *Les Aveugles* at the Fred Hoffman Gallery in Santa Monica are the following (generous) comments:

> What is so compelling about this project is its didactic function.
>   (D. Irmas in the Hoffman catalogue)

> All of these cerebral landscapes are emotionally piercing.
>   (B. Weissman in *Artforum*, November 1989)

> In contrast to more theatrically inclined artists, Calle's involvement with the social yields a celebration of the individual.
>   (B. Butler in the *New Art Examiner*, October 1989)

> In short, *The Blind*, with its open empathy for her subjects, seems symptomatic of Calle's growing self-confidence as an artist.
>   (R. Pincus in *Art in America*, October 1989)

The question that necessarily follows is this: why is it that when deaf artists use sign language in their art or blind artists engage in the tactile or auditory, their work is seen as a cliché; but when sighted, hearing artists appropriate the bodies and thoughts of the disabled their work is applauded as a magnanimous gesture?

Yours,

Joseph

Dear Sophie,

Language, which seems to be the locus here, keeps coming back to me: yours, mine, that of the blind. We mingle our selves, our voices; this room doesn't know passiveness. Perhaps unintentionally, language keeps intruding, asserting itself, taking control. It was Rousseau and Condillac who explained with a sense of irresolvable resolve the humanizing role of language in our lives, how it both makes and unmakes us, defines and dedefines what is around us—even, it seems, what one cannot see, what one cannot hear. It strikes me with a certain acuteness how a number of textual "images" of beauty began as language and remain as language, projected by the seeing on the unseeing:

> *I'm told* white is beautiful

> Green is beautiful. Because every time I like something, *I'm told* it's green

> The sea must be beautiful too. *They tell me* it is blue and green and that when the sun reflects in it, it hurts your eyes

It is easy to tell disabled people what they are missing; much more difficult to listen to, and understand, what they have. Deafness, as Victor Hugo said, is an illness of the mind, not the ears.

Yours,

Joseph

Dear Sophie,

Essentially the matter at hand is difference, or, more precisely, alterity. History is filled with examples of desire to relate to the other in some configuration: to experience the other, possess it, control it. It is, almost ironically, a way of learning more about ourselves, of seeing how we fit into the grand scheme of being— the endless taxonomy of differences that we are forever trying to map, order, and organize into convenient compartments of knowledge. If it were only so simple, Sophie! But of course, it isn't. And it is not always quite the gesture of disinterested benevolence that it seems to be. Difference implies a degree of dispossession; it implies someone else is simultaneously what we want to be and what we fear to be. We want to touch this experience of difference, but we also want to do this from the safe distance of our own identity. We cannot quite forsake who we are to become someone else. We presume that to close our eyes is to experience blindness, or to sleep is to experience death—yet we know that we do not, can not, abandon the sense of self in these endeavors; we cannot "unknow" ourselves as individuals. The imagination, or as Keats might have it, the inmagination, cannot wholly enter into the consciousness of the other, cannot actually become the other. Empathy is an illusion, not a truth: the chameleon may change colors to blend in with its surroundings but it does not become those surroundings.

Yours,

Joseph

Dear Sophie,

Have you ever seen Eadweard Muybridge's nineteenth-century photographs of humans and animals in motion? If you look closely at the serial photographs of people walking, particularly those of disabled people, you might notice among all of them that the idea of "walking" is a generalization for human locomotion—of moving one's body from point A to point B using nothing more than one's own physiological reality. Whether the person is a young child or a young man, a woman with multiple cerebro-spinal sclerosis or a young boy with double amputation of the thighs (Muybridge photographed all of these people), there is no way to define normalcy except through the abstract idea of locomotion: everyone gets from A to B, and that is what is supremely important—not the fact that they get there in different ways.

What one discovers from this is a general idea about difference. As Paul Souriau observed in *The Aesthetics of Movement* (first published in 1889), movement is a product of physiology (or "organic structure"): there is no "normal" body and concomitant movement, but rather an array of differences that reflect themselves in different movements. What is normal is the fact that locomotion is generally possible and that the body will adapt itself to its available resources, exhaust them if necessary, to ensure this possibility—most remarkably—or I should say *un*remarkably—in the case of the double amputee. It is for the same reason that one can argue that speech is not normal to humans, but the basis of speech is—language—and the brain will find another means to produce language in those for whom speech is not possible. Even Rousseau thought of this in his *Essay on the Origin of Language*, struggled with it, but did not have the sort of proof that sign languages of the Deaf offer us today. Thus what is normal is not defined by references to static physiology, but by a dynamic physiology, by the presence of difference. Like atoms spinning off and repelling each other, the marks of difference are ironic formants: at once threatening the collapse of order, they also sustain order. It is only by virtue of differences that we are able to discriminate, it is only by virtue of otherness that language itself is possible: for what is language but the compounding of a finite set of phonological differences into an infinite set of utterances?

> Yours,
>
> Joseph

Dear Sophie,

A short recommended reading list in physiological otherness:

Harlan Lane, *The Mask of Benevolence*
John Hull, *Touching the Rock*
Georges Canguilhem, *The Normal and the Pathological*

Happy reading.

> Yours,
>
> Joseph

Dear Sophie,

Saturday, March 23rd; I am here again in this room, here again among the blind and Sophie Calle. I am surrounded by your signature, yet I do not know who Sophie Calle really is, or who, for that matter, the author of this work really is. The advertisements read "Sophie Calle" but I am inclined to feel that the real artist in this room is not Sophie Calle but the blind themselves, for it is they who do what the artist must necessarily do: find beauty where others do not presume it to be. It is something not unique to the blind with whom Sophie Calle met and talked, but with all blind people, all disabled people, all of us, everyone—even, perhaps, Sophie Calle.

Art historians and contemporary critics are fond of saying that we now live in an age when the ontological distinctions between art and life are necessarily blurred; yet, at the same time, we seem unwilling to acknowledge art that makes no claim to itself as art, but modestly assumes the position of being whatever it finds itself being. Duchamp, it has been claimed, changed the rules by making the everyday object an object of art. The challenge today is to turn this around: to admire the everyday object or the ordinary person precisely because they are not art, and don't care to be.

I'm afraid of my own voice. What, Sophie, have I said?

Yours,

Joseph

Dear Sophie,

There's something more than just a little bit engaging about how the idea of living can itself take on an aesthetic identity, how the *act* of living can supplant the mere object as an aesthetic ideal. At the present moment in cultural history we are facing the end of a century of objecthood, the end of a period in which (particularly during the 1980s) the art object became an object of physically and economically aggrandized proportions. To dismiss this art is not a sign of mere disaffection or residual Marxism; it is instead an act of turning, a gesture toward a certain kind of heretofore unacknowledged unpretentiousness where art is defined by a sincere sense of purpose, by a desire to be everything except this fiction we call art itself. It is, surely, not the only kind of art there is or will be, but it is an art germane, not ancillary, to our contemporary cultural consciousness. Perhaps this is what you yourself are trying to say in *Les Aveugles*. If so, it is a beautiful failure.

Yours,

Joseph

Dear Sophie,

April 17th. I am back, again. The faces, the voices now familiar, a family almost. I give the texts more time now, more space, and as I walked into the gallery today I found myself attracted at once to the blue Braille text of Claude Jauniere. Of all the photographs of objects, reliefs, places, and people which constitute your hermeneutic exercise, it is the Braille text which most belongs here, yet flattened as a photograph it somehow contradicts itself, an oxymoron even. Looking closer—and I must look closer because this text, made to be touched, to be read, is sealed behind glass—I find that this icon of the blind alphabet has been mounted upside down.

Yours,

Joseph

Dear Sophie,

I have double-checked, triple-checked, quadruple-checked the placement of Jauniere's Braille text: upside-down, upside-down, it keeps echoing in my eyes. As I walk up to it, look closely, and step back again, again and again, the visitors to the gallery stare at me, try to comprehend my incomprehension. Surely this is unintentional; yet to call it a "mistake" does not redeem it from my consciousness, where I carry it to a cafe for coffee.

A year ago an acquaintance sent me a postcard, one of a series of *Traffic Signs for the Hearing Impaired* by the painter Martin Wong. In areas frequented by deaf people, particularly near schools for the deaf, America has a tradition of putting up street signs to alert motorists. The signs, normally black lettering on a yellow background, are straightforward and succinct: "Deaf Pedestrians"; "Deaf Child"; "Deaf Children." Wong's postcard showed an attempt to present bilingual texts by spelling "School for Deaf" in both English and the Deaf fingerspelling alphabet. I'm sending you a copy. My acquaintance, an artist herself, thought I would be pleased by this small act of cultural sharing, and at first I was. But when I looked closely at the postcard I noticed that both "f"s had been made wrongly: rather than the thumb and index finger making contact, as they would in a properly configured "f", Wong depicted the thumb in contact with the pinky—the number "6". Instead of saying "School for Deaf" the sign thus said "School 6or Dea6."

The coffee consoles me. Jauniere's Braille text upside-down. This "f" that is not an "f". Not mere mistakes, but misplaced desire.

Yours,

Joseph

Dear Sophie,

April 30th. According to the *New York Gallery Guide, Les Aveugles* has closed, but according to the artworks on the walls of the gallery it continues. The sixth week now. I do not stay long today: the comfort of familiar faces and familiar voices betrays my discomfort.

In the galleries I am genuinely surprised by the presence of traces of the lives of disabled people: enlarged Braille texts, paintings that incorporate codified messages in the Deaf fingerspelling alphabet, sign language tattoos. The disabled seem to be everywhere in the galleries today, but only as subjects, the ordinariness of their lives framed and mounted for those who find it unordinary, "aesthetic," perhaps even strange.

To describe this activity as "appropriation" does not say enough. Couched within this quintessentially postmodern term is a desire to make something one's own, an audacity to assume that we can transpose our selves to another state of being, or to some identity unique to another. The idea of theft is natural when it is unconsciously done within an intertextual matrix—every utterance necessarily steals something—but conscious theft is measured by its consequences, by those who are violated. The question is how far we can take the idea of appropriation, how willfully—or ruefully—we can make it serve our own needs at the expense of others. There is an unspoken line at which appropriation becomes a form of human violence, a point at which theft is transgressed by assault on the human psyche: the point at which appropriation becomes expropriation.

Yours,

Joseph

Dear Sophie,

I am beginning to think of you as a social archaeologist, as one who excavates the shards of human existence, makes notes, photographs, and so on. No scruples, no pettish qualms—truth only.
But whose truth?

Yours,

Joseph

Dear Sophie,

Why is it that I absolutely fail to see any charm or redeeming value in Sam Messer's use of fingerspelling in his paintings? A friend argued that I should at least feel grateful that he brings attention to sign language, and perhaps I should. But what kind of attention is brought to bear here—what perception about sign language, what insights does it offer? The texts are ambiguous, as perhaps they should be: one enters, decodes, and confronts a transcription: "Stop. Listen. Look. Hell Hurts."
Perhaps my problem is with the painting's lifeless two-dimensionality—a travesty of the three-dimensional dynamics of sign language. When fingerspelling is printed as a code, it becomes,

like other writing, inescapably linear: it must be chased by the eye. It is not the mere unnaturalness of this format that is troublesome, but the implication that, by decoding the message, people might be led to think that they are using sign language, when in fact they are doing no more than exercising a simple transcription code: there is no morphology here, no syntax, no movement; the dynamic aspect, the "movement envelope," is lost altogether.

No language, then, but merely the residue of language, a trace of its existence. Like Martin Wong's street signs, Messer's paintings become mere clichés, tokens of familiarity. I do not think, however, that this is the consequence of their being able to hear, but because they are outsiders, attracted more to the ostensibly sequined surface of deafness than the raw undercurrents of the deaf psyche. Even deaf artists are themselves subject to this failure, as is Morris Broderson, who, like Wong and Messer, has a predilection for using fingerspelled texts. One Los Angeles reviewer (Kristine McKenna in the *Los Angeles Times*, 5 December 1986) described Broderson's work as "the kind of stuff you might find adorning the walls of a 12-year-old girl with very bad taste." Frightful criticism, but justified.

From this lesson we might extract two morals: one, that physiology is not the sole criterion for cultural consciousness, and two, a sign cannot exist, cannot mean in a socially meaningful way, apart from the body.

Yours,

Joseph

Dear Sophie,

The paintings by McWilliams and Messer, like your own *Les Aveugles*, lead to a question about the privilege of voices: who "owns" Braille, who "owns" sign language, who has a right to the insights, the mindsights, of the deaf and the blind?

The question itself, though outwardly simple, does not easily engage an answer. Revisionist views of modernism's appropriation of African and Asian mythologies tend to chastise the condescension inherent in the activity (the notion of "primitivism,"

for example) while acknowledging the aesthetic objects that resulted from this cultural interaction—say, Picasso's *Les
Demoiselles*—and the new directions they made possible. This revisionist paradigm can also be found in critical artworks like those
of Fred Wilson, where there is an overt, almost unforgiving critique of Western expropriation of foreign cultures, the museum
being seen as a kind of cultural keyhole. The desire to gaze also
embraces mass-produced objects for Western consumption. If
you browse through the ubiquitous flea markets in Europe, you
can find in shoeboxes old postcards of the people of North
Africa entitled *Scènes et Types*, the Tunisian and Moroccan
women's uniqueness being measured by their jewelry and their
exposed breasts. These cards are not of the tradition of the
risqué (although in contemporary postcard catalogues and auc-
tion lists they are grouped with the risqué), but instead attempt
to proclaim their innocence exploring and marketing cultural
differences. Even Fred Wilson cannot undo the history of muse-
ology without himself becoming a part of that museological context, or without engaging in the use of the same cultural objects
that, as a critique, look manifestly more uncomfortable in a commercial gallery like Gracie Mansion or Metro Pictures than they
do in a museum.

Thus it would probably be wrong to say that the Deaf "own"
sign languages or that the blind own Braille. Yet it would not be
wrong to say that the Deaf and the blind deserve the autonomy
of self-determination, and each excursion made into their cultural territory is subject to critical veracity—it will be looked at,
scrutinized even, by those for whom it is a part of their everyday
lives. Transgressions are severely challenged because they evoke
myths which disability communities have strived for a long time
to eradicate. Most of these myths focus on the illusion of normalcy, the desire of able-bodied people to make the disabled appear normal so that they are less different, less visible in social
and educational domains. Both sign language and Braille, being
arbitrary semiotic codes (one a natural language; the other an
alphabet surrogate) tend to mark their difference in such a way
that it is either aggrandized for the sake of this difference (as in
the work of McWilliams and Messer), or it is repressed because
the difference offends the sense of normalcy in the human community—the same sort of repressive activity that contributes to

the fact that most schools for the deaf and blind, like mental institutions, have been located in rural environments.

Yours,

Joseph

Dear Sophie,

A troubling thought strikes me: who am I to adjudicate the possession of cultural identity? I am embarrassed to think that the postcards I write might be seen as an accretion of warnings from the ubiquitous Culture Police. Am I doing something so low? Who is this Joseph Grigely anyhow? Why does he pronounce so many sentences (both utterances and judgments) upon the work of Sophie Calle? Why is he so obsessed with one solitary installation—*Les Aveugles*?

Perhaps if the history of the disabled were not so static, repetitive, and maligned with stereotypes this would not be necessary; one always feels less comfortable having to react to others than to act on one's own inner impulses. But all art, like all writing, is essentially a conflation of action and reaction, and *Les Aveugles* occupies a very distinct intertextual place among two histories: that of the disabled and that of postmodernism. I am reading these histories, reading into them, and misreading them, as one inevitably will do. But I will not be cajoled by them, and perhaps here we find the source of my resistance and skepticism: I am searching, in a very undeconstructive fashion, for some kind of truth. I do not know what this truth is exactly, so perhaps it is actually truthfulness that I am looking for.

Think of Joseph Grigely not as a person writing these lines but as your conscience coming out of a back room.

Hello, hello!

Yours,

Joseph

Dear Sophie,

Perhaps mere truthfulness is not enough; perhaps what we need here is a hard truth, an upsetting truth, one which can at best be disconcerting and at worst will ultimately be proven wrong. Let me try, anyhow. Listen, Sophie: the presumptuous error of colonialism and the perpetuating error of postcolonialism is a belief that the majority and the minority are static forms. The truth is this: as historically conceived minorities achieve the status of power, they take on the very same qualities as the social institutions they once sought to retract. They become, so to speak, "certified" or "canonized" minorities, perpetuating a myth that is no myth but reality itself: the separation between those who control and those who are controlled. The oppressed become the oppressors.

Nobody, Sophie Calle, can be more "other" than another person. Not you, not I.

Yours,

Joseph

Dear Sophie,

I am getting closer to a theme now. Maybe I was wrong when I first wrote to you and said I had no theoretical locus here. Perhaps there really is. I think it has to do with a topic that hasn't received serious critical discussion: the canonization of difference. The phrase must sound a little bit odd, perhaps even contradictory, but I think that this is a proper moment to bring it up and ask ourselves if in fact it is possible there are marginalized people beyond the margins of the marginalized. Already you can sense that I believe there are. It is not, however, easy to write about the relationship between, say, disability theory and cultural theory, between the disabled as a minority and other canonized minorities and the means by which we define them: race, gender, religion, and national origin. These are familiar phrases because, in America at least, they are used to define difference politically, legislatively, and (in critical discourse) theoretically. But when was the last time a critical journal like *Representations* or *Critical Inquiry* or *Cultural Critique* published an essay about the disabled other—even in special issues devoted to "identity"? Is it because the disabled continue to be patronized as inferiors—that is, as people incapable of participating in contemporary critical discourse? Is it because our signs of difference are just too different to fit into mainstream critical theory? Is it because our presence provokes discomfort that is best kept out of sight—as, historically, has often been the case? Remember those schools for the Deaf and the blind located in rural environments? The very fact that we remain largely absent from mainstream debates about identity and difference, or from the art canon itself, seems to echo the earlier absences felt by now-canonized minorities, who, perhaps understandably, have their territory to protect, their claims of empowerment to guard. Part of the problem, I think, is that we tend to define too much, categorize too much, and find ourselves trapped by our definitions and categories. If we really think about it, it's hard to define what a "mother" is: In Washington D.C. a series of posters promoting foster parenthood have recently appeared. They picture a middle-aged African-American man surrounded by three children, with the caption: "We need more mothers like him." The poster is an eloquent testimony to the fragility of our preconceptions about stereotyped social roles. What it does so well is get alterity out of theories, onto the streets, and into the public consciousness. We need more posters like that. More critical discourse. And more art.

Yours,

Joseph

Dear Sophie,

Never enough time, is there? Or space. . . .

After eight visits to *Les Aveugles*, after 32 postcards, perhaps it is time to come to an end of my monospondence.

I do not mean to imply that I have exhausted possibilities for continuing. No, not that. An ending is a mere formality, the point at which writing stops, the point at which the writer, as a character, exits from his text.

A friend encourages me to be blunt, straightforward, precise.

Since your face is not available to me, why should my face be available to you?

Perhaps, Sophie, you might some day return what you have taken, might some day undress your psyche in a room frequented by the blind, and let them run their fingers over your body as you have run your eyes over theirs.

Yours,

Joseph

WILLIAM STAFFORD

SAYINGS OF THE BLIND

Feeling is believing.

Mountains don't exist. But their slopes do.

Little people have low voices.

All things, even the rocks, make a little noise.

The silence back of all sound is called "the sky."

There's a big stranger in town called the sun.

    He doesn't speak to us but puts out a hand.

Night opens a door into a cellar—

    you can smell it coming.

On Sundays everyone stands farther apart.

Velvet feels black.

Meeting cement is never easy.

What do they mean when they say night is gloomy?

Edison didn't invent much.

Whenever you wake up it's morning.

Names have a flavor.

BURTON RAFFEL

THE BLINDNESS OF A ROSE

Rose most beautiful I've never seen,
round as flesh, shining like the dawn,
squeezes in the darkness of my eye
(which cannot see) as if it were an ecto-
plasmic camel nearing Heaven, leaning
flushed, full, expectant, down on flat
black plates I've slowly grown accustomed to—
living, warm, petals curled and clinging,
clearly bursting backward into beauty
behind the lines of blindness—a rose that needs
to bloom, wanting waves of savor from
the open air, where opening my eye
only now-familiar nothings are.

J. QUINN BRISBEN

THE CICERONE AT ANTIETAM

for W. S.

A perfect day for imperfect bodies:
The mild sun on the well-ramped walks
And glinting in the creek as the pair
Roll and gimp among memories of bodies
Suddenly shattered by a leadstorm,
Then hacked by quick unsterile
Surgeons with nothing to kill the pain;
How they would envy the cicerone's
Plastic and aluminum knee, his elegant
Cane which blooms into a chair
For rest and close observation,
Also his friend the architect's
Power chair humming subserviently,
Agile beyond the smoke-wreathed dreams
Of those who triaged snapped spines
To death tents and lopped limbs
While cursing and being cursed.

Like McClellan, they have the slows,
Drifting leftward on the union lines
Following the eruptions of death
Through the long day of 17 September 1862;
Hooker assaults Lee's left flank;
He cannot reach the Dunker church;
Nor can they, the reconstructed building
Has too many steps; they lack ability
To deploy bodies where needed, again
Like McClellan; further left they note
No corn in Miller's cornfield;

The sunken road is now on the level;
Sinking his cane the cicerone finds
The shallow fords ignored by Burnside,
Who let his troops be slaughtered by the bridge,
Then got across so late that A. P. Hill
Had marched his troops to the field,
Driving unlucky Burnside back;
Then Lee withdrew, McClellan did not follow;
Upwards of a score of thousand corpses rotted,
One more bloody compounding of errors.

The architect asks: "So who won?
McClellan lost more men, but then
He had more men to lose, Lee had
The field but had to go back home,
McClellan should have pursued but did not.
Lincoln pretended the stalemate was a win,
Although he fired McClellan, then issued
The Emancipation Proclamation, a very
Tentative thing on a shaky base."

The cicerone sees their wives
Approaching laden with a trove
And eager to move on; he knows
There is no ending on the surface
Of a sphere, nor in time moving all
At the rate of one minute per minute,
The past receding into warp and blur,
The future forever beyond our kenning.
Anyhow he speaks: "There is no victory
When so many die. Maybe Lincoln,
Everybody's favorite rail-splitting
Corporation lawyer and bloody saint,
Our master of myth and spin control,
Did well to use this mess as fulcrum
To move a nation to a good end;
You and I are joined for a good end, too,
Using what is at hand, which is all we have.
Come, no more time to rake this over,
Though it has been a good and useful pause,
It is time to roll the movement on."

CAROL POORE

"BUT ROOSEVELT COULD WALK": ENVISIONING DISABILITY IN GERMANY AND THE UNITED STATES

> It is inconceivable that the ever-progressive FDR would be pleased to have a memorial that denies his greatest political achievement: evading the physical barriers and social biases of an ableist society in order to lead the nation out of its darkest hours.[1]

1. "But Roosevelt Could Walk"

On November 25, 1991, the German weekly news magazine *Der Spiegel* featured an article on the prominent Christian Democratic politician Wolfgang Schäuble, who was widely regarded as the most likely conservative successor to Chancellor Helmut Kohl. The cover photo, captioned "Will he hold up?" showed Schäuble seated in his wheelchair in a thoughtful pose, while another photo placed him in the awkwardly posed center of a group of his cabinet colleagues (Figs. 1 and 2). Schäuble, the Minister of the Interior, had been shot in an assassination attempt in October of 1990, shortly after German reunification, and as a result his legs were paralyzed. Now back on the job and using a wheelchair, he was about to assume the chairmanship of the conservative Christian Democratic party (CDU/CSU) fraction in the German parliament. The significance of this new political position was that it gave him a great deal of leverage in being selected by his party in the future as its candidate for chancellor, which *Der Spiegel* commented on in this article as follows:

> After Kohl has finished off all his opponents within his party, it could seem as though he is making a mockery of Schäuble's

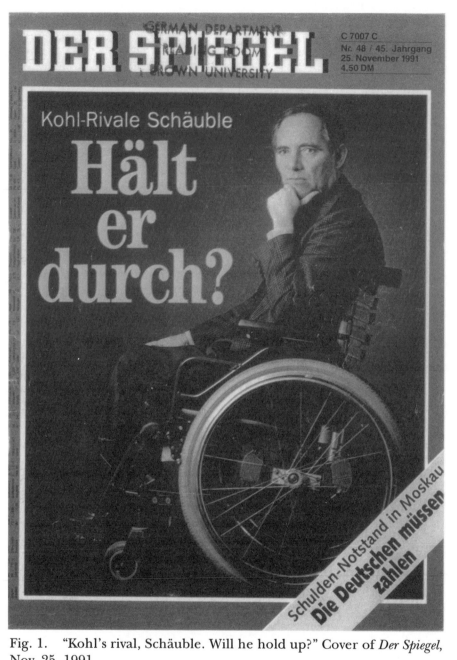

Fig. 1.   "Kohl's rival, Schäuble. Will he hold up?" Cover of *Der Spiegel*, Nov. 25, 1991.

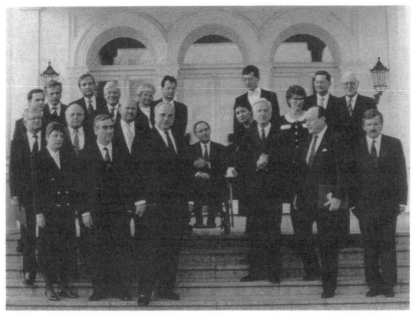

Fig. 2. Wolfgang Schäuble seated in the center of Helmut Kohl's cabinet. *Der Spiegel*, Nov. 25, 1991.

possible rivals by setting up a paralytic as his potential successor to the chancellorship. Kohl talks about the example of U.S. President Franklin D. Roosevelt, who, Kohl says, also governed his country from a wheelchair. The important difference: Roosevelt, who contracted polio, could walk unaided (though with crutches). Schäuble is paralyzed from the third vertebra down, and the wheelchair is his irrevocable fate.[2]

Yet, of course, the wheelchair was also Roosevelt's "irrevocable fate." The fact that the leading German news magazine could present such an erroneous description of the U.S. president more than forty-five years after his death only testifies to the enduring legacy of Roosevelt's efforts to control his public image. While this strategy was entirely necessary during his lifetime in order for him to attain his goals, it also perpetuates misconceptions of the true extent of his disability in popular memory, as the *Spiegel* article shows. Roosevelt and Schäuble are not comparable at all as far as their political stature is concerned—Schäuble is basically a clever, conservative bureaucrat. However, from the instant when he set out to re-enter the German political arena in a wheelchair, depictions of his disability became central to all speculations about whether he was capable of filling the highest political office in Germany. Debate about Schäuble's qualifications has been enmeshed with the images which the German public sees of him, while on this side of the Atlantic, another kind of controversy has arisen in the last few years over the depiction of Roosevelt's disability at the new memorial to him in Washington, D.C. Therefore, juxtaposing the visual images of these two prominent political figures provides a way to focus on changing perceptions and symbolic meanings of disability in the United States and Germany.

Historians have documented in detail the lengths to which Roosevelt went, almost always with the cooperation of the press, to present himself to the public as non-disabled after he contracted polio in 1921 at the age of 39.[3] The extent of his paralysis was such that he was only able at most to take a few precarious steps alone using braces and crutches, and he in fact used a wheelchair from then on. Yet Roosevelt was also wealthy and a well-established politician, having served as Secretary of the Navy and having already been nominated for Vice President at the Democratic National Convention in 1920. Certainly the fact that he was so well-known and successful made it easier for him to re-enter politics and be accepted as a viable candidate, in spite of speculation about his physical condition. After several years of convalescence and rehabilitation, Roosevelt was elected governor of New York in 1928 and re-elected in 1930. He was elected to his first term as president in 1932 and died in office shortly into his fourth term in April of 1945 in Warm Springs, Georgia, at the "Little White House" close to the treatment center for polio which he had founded.

In 1924, Roosevelt nominated Al Smith for president at the Democratic National Convention, and this was his first major appearance in public after having polio. From the outset, he was determined to avoid the stigma of being seen in public in a wheelchair, with all its associations of invalidism and incompetence. At this convention, he was photographed using crutches for the only time. Later on, his physical therapist reported him describing his goal like this: "I'll walk without crutches. I'll walk into a room without scaring everybody half to death. I'll stand

easily enough in front of people so that they'll forget I'm a cripple."[4] From then on, Roosevelt's project of presenting himself to
the public as non-disabled was essentially a two-pronged strategy:
first, to exude the aura of self-confidence and authority which
was expected from leading men in politics; and second, to avoid
disrupting visual expectations of bodily normalcy. Accordingly,
the two images of Roosevelt which are probably the most enduring are his trademark big smile with the jaunty cigarette holder
and his head tilted back, and the photographs of Roosevelt
seated between Stalin and Churchill at Yalta.

Any arbitrary selection of images from the press shows the
care Roosevelt took to avoid making his disability the distracting
focal point. When he stood, he generally either held a lectern
the way that any other speaker might, or he gripped the arm of a
companion and used one gentlemanly cane, all the while wearing pants cut extra long in order to hide his braces. When sitting, he appeared in ordinary poses: behind the wheel of his car,
busy at his desk, or sitting with other politicians such as in the
Yalta picture. There are only a few private photos researchers
have uncovered in the Roosevelt archives which give more accu-
rate impressions of the extent of his disability. Of these, only two
photos actually show him using a wheelchair, including a very
tender one with his dog Fala and an employee's young daughter
at Hyde Park (Fig. 3).

If attitudes toward disability were so negative that Roosevelt
felt compelled to control his public image in this way in order to
have the life and career that he wanted, it is not at all obvious
why the press went along for the most part with strict regulations
from the White House prohibiting photos showing him using
crutches or a wheelchair. Yet with very few exceptions coming
from the ranks of his most adverse critics, there appears to have
been a kind of gentleman's agreement between Roosevelt and
the press not to make an issue of his disability and not to focus
on it visually. A crucial factor here, in contrast to a later politician such as Schäuble, is that Roosevelt lived in the pre-television
age, at a time when visual images were much less ubiquitous and
much easier to control—and also during the heyday of radio, a
medium where the stigma of visible physical disability dropped
away and which Roosevelt used with great virtuosity. Since he was
already proven in the political arena, he was perhaps granted the
benefit of the doubt when he set out to re-enter politics. And

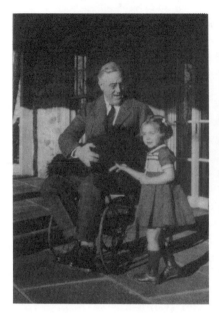 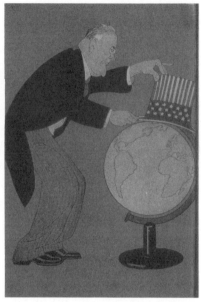

Fig. 3. (left) One of two known photographs of Roosevelt seated in his wheelchair (at Hyde Park). Fig. 4. (right) Nazi cartoon of Roosevelt. Back cover of Martin Pase (pseud. of Ernest Pasemann), *Roosevelts Reden und Taten im Scheinwerfer der Presse und der Karikatur* (Berlin: Lühe, 1941).

after he became president, he used his communication skills to create a generally cordial relationship with the Washington press corps, so that there are records of photographers voluntarily destroying negatives which might have shown too revealing images of his disability. Perhaps, too, as long as Roosevelt was doing a more than competent job in office—first in responding to the Great Depression and then as Commander-in-Chief during the war—members of the press were willing to go along with the idea that the President of the United States was by definition strong and authoritative, and to continue producing this image. Even political cartoonists, who traditionally seize upon the slightest deviation from the norm as material for their satiric exaggeration, never portrayed Roosevelt's disability but focused on other features, most notably, his huge grin and the cigarette holder.

And in cartoons which depicted his entire body, he was always portrayed as non-disabled (untrue) and active (true).

The presentation and depiction of Roosevelt's disability in his post-1921 political career is particularly entangled, then. On the one hand, Roosevelt knew that physical disability—a body which did not correspond to the norm and which perhaps needed technical or mechanical aids and the assistance of others to function—was an automatic disqualification for public life, let alone for the highest political office. On the other hand, if the fact of disability could be concealed and a non-disabled image presented to the public, a man of Roosevelt's intellect, wealth, and connections could succeed in attaining his goals. In spheres outside the fishbowl of Washington politics, Roosevelt reacted to the experience of disability by identifying with it and becoming an advocate in certain ways. Most notably, he established the Georgia Warm Springs Foundation and spent time socializing with other polio patients there; he helped create the National Foundation for Infantile Paralysis (commonly known as the "March of Dimes") which raised money for needy polio patients and for research on developing a polio vaccine; and on at least one occasion, he visited a hospital ward for disabled veterans in his wheelchair.[5] In the arena of politics, Roosevelt's concealment of his disability and the press's cooperation reflected a view of the disabled body as stigmatizing, shameful, and as a physical marker of weakness of intellect and character. Yet the consciousness of this concealment also indicates a knowledge that these views were becoming increasingly outdated in the modern world—though the benefits of acting upon this knowledge were generally only available to the most exceptional individuals in the days before disability rights perspectives took hold.

Even though Roosevelt's disability was caused by disease and was not congenital, it is nevertheless a striking fact that a president with a visibly imperfect body was elected for four terms during a period when eugenics was thriving in many Western countries, including the U.S., and when eugenic thinking led to its most terrible results in Nazi Germany. It might be logical to think, then, that the Nazi press would have seized upon Roosevelt's physical condition as convenient material for anti-American propaganda. Yet, as in the U.S., pictorial images of Roosevelt in the Nazi press during the years of his presidency hardly ever showed his disability, although here a different dynamic was at work. A book published in Germany in 1941 entitled *Roosevelt's Speeches and Actions in the Spotlight of the Press and of Political Cartoons (Roosevelts Reden und Taten im Scheinwerfer der Presse und der Karikatur)* collected cartoons from the German and foreign press which often used hateful antisemitic images to depict Roosevelt as a puppet of the Jews, as a warmonger, or as a failure with his New Deal, but his disability is hardly evident.[6] For example, the book's front cover features Roosevelt admiring his mirror reflection as a Jew. Other cartoons show Roosevelt and Churchill as puppets of the Jews, a blind Roosevelt being led by a Jew (this from a U.S. pro-Nazi newspaper), and Roosevelt being ridden, and thus controlled, by Jews in a "Jewish kindergarten." Another group of cartoons combines antisemitic imagery with attacks on America's supposed belligerence and desire for world domination. The back cover shows a standing Roosevelt putting Uncle Sam's hat over the entire globe (Fig. 4), and another cartoon transforms his famous toothy grin into a mouthful of bombs. One particularly loathsome cartoon depicts Roosevelt holding a barely visible cane while supervising Jews who are torturing the American people and preparing for war. Finally, the magazine of satire called *Kladderadatsch* published the only cartoon I know which shows Roosevelt with two canes, headed down the "path of Wilson" into war (Fig. 5). It appears that the image of Roosevelt's disability in the Nazi press did not change in any significant way as the war progressed. Later, in newspapers such as *Das Reich*, there were relatively few cartoons depicting Roosevelt, since the U.S. was usually portrayed as an ugly Uncle Sam, along with Britain's John Bull and France's Marianne.

Undoubtedly there was a certain amount of knowledge abroad, including in Nazi Germany, about Roosevelt's physical condition, although it is not so clear whether the extent of his limitations was recognized. One graphic statement was made by Mussolini on the occasion of a speech by Roosevelt that Italy's fascist leader especially disliked: "Never in the course of history has a nation been guided by a paralytic. There have been bald kings, fat kings, handsome and even stupid kings, but never kings who, in order to go to the bathroom and the dinner table, had to be supported by other men."[7] In Germany, comments on Roosevelt's disability seemed to focus mainly on the supposed connection between physical illness and mental or emotional condition. The Nazi editor of the above-mentioned book of po-

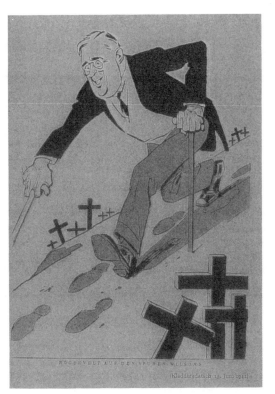

Fig. 5. "Roosevelt going down Wilson's path." Nazi cartoon from *Kladderadatsch,* June 15, 1941, reprinted in Pase (see Fig. 4).

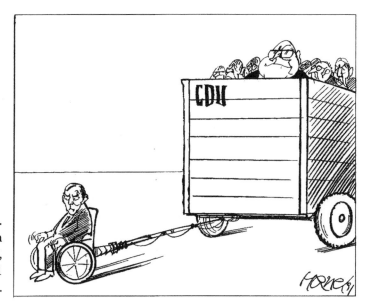

Fig. 6. Cartoon from *Der Spiegel,* Sept. 23, 1991 (page 20).

litical cartoons, for example, referred to FDR's bout with polio by saying that "After a few years his affliction improved so that he was able to return to the political arena in 1928, but the struggle with his illness not only increased his high self-esteem, but also increased his desire to be active in a very dangerous way."[8] And he went on to say that it was probably possible to understand Roosevelt's mentality only by realizing that he was "a physically broken person who is constantly venting his hysteria."[9]

Hitler himself referred to Roosevelt as manipulated by the Jews, as wealthy (in contrast to Hitler's supposedly impoverished origins), and as insane. Yet even in his final monologues, which record his more informal conversations, he made no reference to Roosevelt's physical condition. Instead, he emphasized repeatedly his belief that Roosevelt was mentally unstable, as in the following passage from March 23, 1942, where he attributed the hysteria over the "War of the Worlds" radio broadcast to Roosevelt's unsettling influence:

> Roosevelt is insane, as a professor already explained years ago. He rushes chaotically from Washington to his estate out of fear of being bombed, rushes back, and so on. His press statements also show that the man is insane. He's making his whole country hysterical, the way he's going. How could it be possible otherwise that a panic could break out among reasonable people in Chicago because of a radio play about Martians landing there.[10]

Again, it is unclear what Hitler and other Nazi leaders knew about the extent of Roosevelt's disability. It could be that Roosevelt's policy of appearing as non-disabled as possible in public was effective in limiting the extent of knowledge abroad about his inability to walk. It could also have been the case that Nazi leaders and their press knew more about his physical condition but chose not to depict it. If the latter was true, this would confirm the general approach the Nazis took to depicting people with disabilities, especially those who were the objects of their "euthanasia" and sterilization campaigns. Rather than targeting such people for ridicule or hatred through distorting caricatures or drawings,[11] Nazi ideologues and medical professionals attempted to win over the sympathy of the public for eliminating the "unfit" by using more "scientific" depictions. These included, above all, photographs of patients in mental hospitals and children with birth defects, along with similar propaganda films and mathematical examples of how the nation's resources were being wasted on such people.[12] It is easy to imagine that if photographs of Roosevelt in a wheelchair or in other situations where his physical weakness was readily apparent had been widely circulating, the Nazi press would have made use of these as opportunities to give a negative, seemingly objective portrayal of their great adversary.

2. "Will He Hold Up?"

More than half a century after the longest-serving president devised his strategy for success, the development of the mass media and above all of television makes it impossible for public figures to hide a visible disability in the same way. And, more positively put, it has been the great achievement of modern civil rights movements to disentangle physical characteristics and mental ability from automatic assignments of social status. Consequently, since Roosevelt's time, consciousness has also grown that there should be no compelling reasons for hiding disability, for trying to "pass" in the able-bodied world. Today, the case of Wolfgang Schäuble is especially interesting, because he is not only a prominent politician with a disability, but also an object of media attention in the country which tried during the Nazi period to create the homogeneous national racial community ("Volksgemeinschaft") by eliminating all manner of "deviants" from public life.[13] Visual images of Schäuble and of other people with disabilities in Germany today can thus be taken as one barometer of the extent to which deviation from concepts of a physical or mental norm may be tolerated in this country, which has undergone such extreme political and cultural ruptures in the twentieth century.

The visual images of Schäuble in photographs in German news magazines, in political cartoons, and on German television differ from those of Roosevelt in that Schäuble is always shown using his wheelchair except for a few family shots. The wheelchair is a fact of his life, an extension of his body, and there is no attempt to hide it at all. I would propose that these images float back and forth between two poles, which Schäuble has challenged most recently by going on the offensive as a "cripple." On the one hand are those which—consciously or unconsciously—dredge up old stereotypes to show him literally as a "foreign body," as a disturbance and disruption of the well-ordered, normative physical world. These images provoke discomfort in the viewer, making Schäuble into the object of the stare by showing him sitting while others are standing and sitting in unusual situations, or by using captions which draw attention to his anomalous physical condition. Perhaps the best illustration of such a perception is the image of Schäuble perched awkwardly at the top of the steps among the rest of Kohl's Cabinet, which makes it seem impossible that such a person could ever "fit" into this political world.[14] Numerous photographs show Schäuble in the wheelchair while other politicians stand beside it or in positions which emphasize his isolation. One of the most distasteful of these appeared in the illustrated magazine *Stern* (a kind of German *Life*) on August 20, 1992. Captioned "Unapproachable, Uncanny, Relentless," it shows Schäuble in a row with other people who are only visible from the waist down. This article demonstrated that some of the oldest and most damaging stereotypes about people with disabilities are still current by attributing Schäuble's hard-nosed brand of politics to his supposed bitterness over being excluded from the "normal" world and claiming that there was something "uncanny" about the "iron strength of will" with which he pursued his goals.

A second group of photographs, however, treats Schäuble's disability in a more matter-of-fact way by not making the wheelchair into the main personal or political feature overriding all his other traits. There are numerous images which show him sitting and conversing with Kohl and other politicians or addressing Parliament in his wheelchair from the podium. The ways in which preconceived attitudes influence the interpretation of disability come out particularly clearly in the use of one photo which shows Schäuble reaching for the microphone in Parliament. *Stern* captioned this picture "The bully's return," while *Der Spiegel* called it "A hard road."

Political cartoons featuring Schäuble always show his wheelchair, in contrast to those depicting Roosevelt, and also reflect these ambivalent perceptions of disability. In some, the wheelchair is simply a fact but is not central to the political point being made. In others, the perception of disability is inextricably entangled in the political statement, as several cartoons from *Der Spiegel* illustrate. These all center around the fact that Kohl and his Christian Democratic Party had begun to have more and more difficulties in the early 1990s due to the political and economic problems associated with reunification. The first, with no caption, shows a diminutive Schäuble with his wheelchair hitched to a large wagon labeled "CDU" containing Kohl and other politicians (Fig. 6). Is his party pinning all its hopes on him? Is this an impossible task for the disabled politician? The second, captioned "Getting out of the critical zone," shows a clearly overburdened Schäuble zooming along in his wheelchair, almost crushed by Kohl, who is sitting on his lap. Will Schäuble be the one to save Kohl? Is it a sad commentary on the state of Kohl's ruling coalition that it has to be rescued by a man in a wheelchair? The third, captioned "The miracle weapon," shows Schäuble as an archer in his wheelchair, leading the forces of the conservative party out into battle. Is he hopelessly inadequate to the task; is he a courageous fighter; or is he simply setting out to accomplish the political tasks at hand?[15]

The ambivalence of these views of disability also comes through in the letters to the editor which reacted to *Der Spiegel*'s cover story on Schäuble. Some readers viewed his disability as an automatic disqualification for political office, stating, for example, that he was being coddled as Kohl's potential successor out of misplaced sympathy for his misfortune, or that there was something mentally unstable in his continuing obsession with political power. One reader captured this point of view in a nutshell by stating: "Now Kohl has picked somebody whom no one can compete with out of simple decency—even though it must be obvious to every clearly thinking person that a man with such a severe handicap as Schäuble's is physically simply not up to the stress of being chancellor." Others criticized *Der Spiegel* for focusing so heavily on Schäuble's disability in the article and called for a more objective appraisal. As one letter noted: "If Dr. Schäuble holds up, that will depend only on his politics, and not on the wheelchair portrayed on your cover. In any case, it is not helpful to the approximately eight million disabled in the Federal Republic, who make it and hold up anyway, to connect the evaluation of his politics to his physical disability."[16] Such statements, along with the fact that Schäuble has continued to hold on to his influential position, indicate an increase in liberal attitudes in Germany, which means an increased ability to tolerate at least a certain amount of difference without moving immediately to exclude or eliminate disturbing deviation.

3. "We Are Also the People"

My choice of words here recalls an earlier time, of course. After all, Roosevelt was able to conceal his impairment and become president, but the majority of people with disabilities at that time were segregated in life-diminishing ways: concealed from the sight of others by being kept at home or in institutions, excluded from the workplace and from public life. This sort of exclusion culminated in efforts to eliminate some groups of people with disabilities altogether during the heyday of eugenics in the first half of the twentieth century, when many countries, including the United States, developed involuntary sterilization programs.[17] Eugenic thinking had the most murderous consequences under the Nazi regime, when between 300,000 and 500,000 people with various disabilities and illnesses were sterilized involuntarily and about 120,000 people with mental illnesses and other disabilities were killed under the so-called "euthanasia" program.[18] As one facet of the Nazis' racist agenda, these criminal acts were aimed at creating a more homogeneous national racial community through the elimination of those held to be inferior in their genetic makeup, although the net for capturing so-called "undesirables" came to be cast ever wider.

The trauma of this governmentally institutionalized violence still resurfaces at times in the discourse about disability in Germany today, shaping debates and actions in certain ways and molding the vocabulary used to describe disability and connect it to other types of difference. The debate over new ethical dilemmas created by advances in medical technology provides the most recent case in point. As in all countries with access to scientific advances, these questions of bioethics center most often around the acceptability of prenatal testing for genetic defects, abortion on the basis of genetic indications, passive or active euthanasia of babies born with severe birth defects and other people in certain extreme situations, and physician-assisted suicide.

What has become known as the "new debate over euthanasia" in Germany—and so implicitly over the "worth of life," a phrase carrying an enormously heavy historical burden[19]—began in the summer of 1989, when Australian philosopher Peter Singer was invited to speak at a European Symposium on "Bioengineering, Ethics, and Mental Disability" in Marburg.[20] On the same tour, he was also invited to give lectures in Dortmund on the topic,

"Do severely disabled newborn infants have a right to life?" and at several other conferences and symposia. Known for his books on animal rights and on questions of practical and applied ethics, Singer had argued that under certain specific conditions it was ethically permissible for physicians to kill infants with severe birth defects.[21] For my purposes here, the exact grounding of his argumentation—which can be characterized as a utilitarian approach remarkably lacking in sensitivity to the complexities of life—is less interesting than the reactions which his scheduled appearances provoked in Germany. The mounting protests against Singer from organizations of people with disabilities, along with other groups such as coalitions against genetic engineering, were so intense that the invitations to him were cancelled for the most part, and one of the conferences where he was scheduled to speak was moved to Holland. Two years later, in May of 1991, at a lecture Singer was scheduled to give at the University of Zürich on animal rights, a group of listeners in wheelchairs staged a protest, stating that they objected to the university inviting such a "notorious advocate of euthanasia to discuss ethical issues." The audience then began to chant "Singer out," and he was prevented from speaking. Since then, protests and even threats of violence have continued to block many public discussions in Germany about these issues.

From the point of view of the protesting individuals and groups, these debates should be prevented at all costs because they are always the first step along the proverbial "slippery slope" which leads to judging some lives to be more "valuable" than others. Those who take this standpoint maintain that even discussing questions such as euthanasia necessarily means questioning the right to life of all people with any kind of disabilities.[22] The most vocal organizations of people with disabilities in Germany appear to support the view that bioethics is quite simply an illegitimate field of inquiry.[23] It is hardly imaginable that there would not be serious disruptions there of a program such as that planned by the U.S. Society for Disability Studies for its spring 1997 meeting, where members of this organization and experts on bioethics considered together the implications for people with disabilities of new developments in human genetics and prenatal diagnosis. In any event, those calling for unfettered debate about these issues in Germany have not made very much headway.

The most perceptive analyses of this stalemate have emphasized the ways in which memory of Nazi crimes continues to
shape these confrontations. For example, in an article published
in Germany's leading weekly newspaper, *Die Zeit*, on October 25,
1991, the philosopher Ernst Tugendhat made a plea for an open
and tolerant debate about euthanasia, maintained that it was
only "in the German-speaking regions that the handicapped
were reacting in such a way," and criticized the irrationality and
lack of differentiations on both sides of the confrontation over
Singer. He attributed this inability to carry on rational debate to
repressed guilt feelings over the Nazi past which still had not
been worked through. According to Tugendhat, this could be
seen by the way people with disabilities instrumentalized knowledge about the murder of "lives unworthy of life" to prevent debate even though they also wanted to be accepted as citizens with
no special privileges (and certainly not the privilege of blocking
freedom of speech). On the other hand, he also criticized universities and other organizations that withdrew their invitations
to Singer as a result of the protests rather than take a chance of
being tainted in any way by association with past crimes.[24]

Certainly memory of the German past is a central factor in
shaping these debates, or better, confrontations. Yet I also think
it important to probe deeper into the reasons existing in the present for what might seem an intransigent standpoint taken by activist organizations of people with disabilities on these issues.
After all, the intensity of marginalization which these groups still
experience is also a force which drives them to take radical positions. Therefore, I would like to comment briefly on tendencies
toward exclusion directed against people with disabilities in Germany, as well as on self-help groups and organizations which
have resisted such pressures in recent years.

On the one hand, in both East and West Germany and then in
the reunified country, people with disabilities have long had access to a range of free or inexpensive social services hardly imaginable in the United States. On the other hand, the provision of
these services without comparable efforts at integration often
seems to have the unintended countereffect of locking people
with disabilities into a cycle of living from welfare payments and
segregating them from "normal" life activities. As in other countries, people with disabilities are excluded from the labor market
to an extent which hardly correlates with their desires and abili-

ties to work. In West Germany, for example, approximately 17% of women and 42% of men with disabilities work at any kind of job, somewhat less than half the percentages for their non-disabled counterparts.[25] With regard to education, an extensive system of special schools exists. In East Germany before 1989, there were no efforts to integrate children with disabilities who needed any kind of accommodations into regular classes. In West Germany, for the past twenty years or so, groups of committed parents and teachers have pushed for mainstreaming, but only with very limited local successes. And predictably, the "special school" is generally a road to a second-class education, to occupational dead ends, and to life as a social misfit.[26] As far as the sphere of personal relationships goes, which is certainly the most difficult to generalize about, a varied picture emerges from autobiographies and first-hand accounts, of people with disabilities who lead full and happy lives and of others who attribute their loneliness and isolation to rejection because of their difference.[27]

Along with these more general tendencies toward separating out people with disabilities from the mainstream of life, which have only been exacerbated by the economic restructuring since reunification, there were several widely noted incidents of violence against people with disabilities in the early 1990s, at the same time that the debate about euthanasia and bioethics was intensifying. For a few years after reunification, especially in 1992 and 1993, violent attacks—some resulting in death—against foreign workers and refugees, as well as instances where concentration camp sites were vandalized and Jewish cemeteries desecrated, spread across both Eastern and Western Germany. Less frequent, but still noticeable enough to be reported on with some prominence in the German and U.S. press, were a number of attacks on people with disabilities.[28] For example, groups of youths described as having neo-Nazi tendencies beat up pupils at a school for deaf children and at an occupational rehabilitation center, and residents of a group home were attacked with stones in a street riot where, according to *Der Spiegel*, "foreigners and handicapped persons were harassed and beaten."[29] The sober weekly *Die Zeit* entitled its article about these incidents "Clubs against Cripples" and veered toward sensationalism by stating: "The handicapped are being insulted, spat upon, beaten. One of their spokesmen fears: 'After the foreigners, it might be the turn of the handicapped. And when the avalanche starts, it's too late.'"[30] And some time later, the same newspaper maintained apodictically in an article about the growth of right-wing organizations in Germany: "More and more young people hate foreigners and the handicapped. They want an authoritarian state."[31]

Here, memory of the past was intertwined with fears of violence in the present. On the one hand, whether out of watchfulness or merely the habit of repeating well-learned paradigms, the reporting on these incidents generally exaggerated the extent of the hostility directed against people with disabilities in their daily lives. On the other, these threatening events were certainly one source for the unyielding, intolerant position that some of Singer's opponents took in the euthanasia debate. Seen in this context, a headline by one of these activists proclaiming that the mood of the day was "Disabled out" (recalling the Nazi cry of "Jews out") was not totally overwrought.[32] And an article in a progressive medical journal was not completely farfetched when it predicted that the increasing material, psychic, and social insecurities of the German population after reunification might cause increasing tendencies toward exclusion of people with disabilities and foreigners.[33] Striking in this entire discussion has been the frequent recurrence of the phrase "foreigners and the handicapped," which recalls a constellation of groups who were marked by National Socialism to be excluded from the healthy body of the national racial community due to their ethnic, racial, genetic, physical, or mental "otherness."

To counteract these tendencies toward violence, people with disabilities in Germany organized self-defense groups and informational activities, and participated in the large candlelight marches which took place in many German cities after the wave of attacks against foreigners (Fig. 7). As in many other countries, people with disabilities have organized themselves in West Germany since the late 1960s in order to provide mutual support, to create ways of speaking out and becoming more visible, and so to gain increased political and social leverage. Generally having the goal of greater social integration, the activities of these groups are similar to ones carried out in the United States, with the important difference that there is as yet no civil rights law in Germany corresponding to the Americans with Disabilities Act. In East Germany before 1989, independent advocacy organizations were prohibited, and so it was only in the winter of

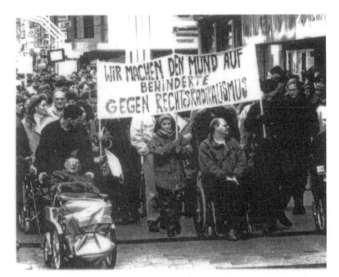

Fig. 7. "We're speaking out. Disabled against right-wing radicalism." *Die Randschau,* Vol. 8, Nr. 1 (March/April 1993), 22.

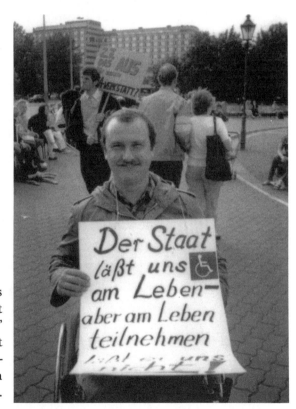

Fig. 8. "The State lets us live, but doesn't let us participate in life." First united East/West demonstration of people with disabilities in Berlin, May 1990.

1989/1990 that East Germans with disabilities became able to speak out publicly about their dissatisfactions and goals.

In May of 1990, a few months before reunification took place, the first united East/West demonstration of people with disabilities and their non-disabled supporters took place in Berlin. The speakers and large variety of groups present give a good idea of the issues Germans with disabilities considered most important at that time. Eastern speakers voiced apprehension over what the coming of West German capitalism and models of health care would mean for them, and some of their demands also reflected the concerns of Westerners. Slogans on banners called for "work for all," questioned whether people with disabilities would be left behind after the imminent currency reform, and called for insurance and attendants for independent living. Yet also, as the group rolled and walked past what had been the East German Parliament, there was a sense of exhilaration over being able to speak out together. Other banners demanded "mobility for the disabled," "no exclusion," and "self-determination, not charity," and proclaimed "Whoever leaves us out violates human rights." One poster declared "The State lets us live, but doesn't let us participate in life" (Fig. 8), while another picked up the slogan from the fall 1989 demonstrations in Leipzig which finally brought down the East German government, to proclaim "We are also the people." In this demonstration, as on other political occasions, the visual images of people with disabilities are ones of diversity and action which dream of a more open and inclusive world. It remains to be seen whether reunified Germany, a society increasingly oriented toward profit and competitive individual performance, will be able to live up to these hopes.

4. "A Cripple as Chancellor?" Schäuble and Roosevelt Revisited

The different ways in which disability is configured in broad public discussions in Germany and the United States today appear strikingly in the most recent press speculations on Schäuble's qualifications to be chancellor and in the controversy over the new Roosevelt Memorial in Washington, D.C. Until Helmut Kohl finally let it be known in April of 1997 that he would run for a fifth term as chancellor, Schäuble was still looked upon as the most likely Christian Democratic candidate, although after Kohl's announcement, some reporters began calling Schäuble

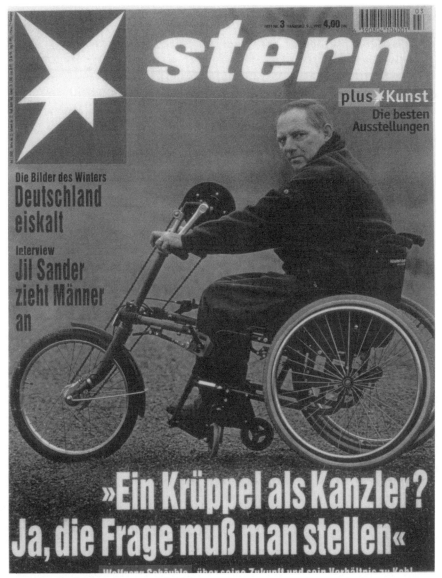

Fig. 9. "'A cripple as Chancellor? Yes, the question must be asked.' Wolfgang Schäuble on his future and his relationship to Kohl." Cover of *Stern*, Jan. 9, 1997.

the "Prince Charles of German politics." In any event, the wheel-chair was an issue which Schäuble was determined to bury once and for all by pursuing the strategy of ruthless openness about his physical condition and appropriating the vocabulary which his opponents had sometimes directed against him. In 1992, for example, *Stern* had quoted unnamed members of Parliament as voicing the thoughts which many people with disabilities often imagine to be lurking underneath superficial politeness: "He's nothing but a head," "He sits in his room like a spider in a web," "He's such an obsessive politician because he can't get anything else out of life."

Schäuble went on the offensive in the January 9, 1997 issue of *Stern*, appearing seated in his three-wheel wheelchair/tricycle on the cover, which quoted him in its headline: "'A Cripple as Chancellor? Yes, the Question Must Be Asked.' Wolfgang Schäuble on His Future and His Relationship to Kohl" (Fig. 9). The magazine's editorial page recalled Roosevelt's example again (correctly this time, in contrast to the earlier *Spiegel* article) and went on in a long interview with Schäuble to report on his health, described as stable, and his close relationship to Kohl, noting that a recent poll had shown that 57% of Germans believed him qualified to be chancellor in spite of his disability. In the next week's issue of the magazine, the editor reported that he had never received as much criticism as for the cover story on Schäuble and printed a sampling of indignant letters. Most readers had failed to notice that the headline was a quote from Schäuble himself, and so they accused *Stern* of tastelessness and gross insensitivity for describing him as a "cripple." A few others chose to focus more on challenging his political qualifications, while only one picked up the old image of disability as a symbol of incompetence, stating: "Why shouldn't a cripple become chancellor? The German people are limping along in a bad way, anyhow. So a chancellor in a wheelchair really fits into the picture well."

The subsequent discussion in the German press about the *Stern* article evaluated it as highly significant for Schäuble's tactics in trying to break two taboos. First, he had successfully stated his interest in becoming Kohl's successor (without being immediately put down by the chancellor himself). Second, by appropriating for himself the negative term "cripple," he had made it more difficult for his political adversaries to take a patronizing approach toward him. Along these lines, for example, *Der Spiegel* stated on February 10, 1997: "Only by constantly breaking taboos can he convince the Germans, who are always curious and torn back and forth between admiration and discomfiture, that his existence as a paraplegic is only marginally different from real life [*sic!*]. . . . The leader of the CDU fraction wants to prove that a politician needs little more for success than a head and arms."

Most striking, I think, in these latest depictions of Schäuble, is the bluntness with which his disability is visualized and described, both by himself and by journalists.[34] The harsh directness of the tone can have both positive and questionable aspects. On the one hand, as one disability rights advocate pointed out, the latest *Stern* cover story can be taken as visualizing the wheelchair/tricycle as expanding the range of possibilities for a disabled person rather than as a limitation, and thus as creating an emancipatory portrait.[35] Furthermore, Schäuble's appropriation for himself of the label "cripple" and the lack of any inhibitions in reporting which speculates about his condition could be said to evidence some refreshing honesty by saying publicly what many people usually keep in the backs of their minds. On the other hand, however, the frequency with which even putatively sympathetic journalists resort to characterizing Schäuble as a man with only a "head and arms" or photographing him in ways which produce images of an overly large wheelchair still appears to contain elements of the belief that there is something fundamentally different, strangely freakish, about disability which separates such a politician from the "normal" world. And as for Schäuble's self-descriptions, these seem more like ploys to advance his political future than positive efforts to associate himself with other people with disabilities. As far as I am aware, he has never lent his support to disability advocacy groups who are working for greater integration.[36] On the contrary, he remains a conservative bureaucrat whose policies, if he ever were elected chancellor, would probably be undesirable and damaging to many people with disabilities who are living on limited incomes. And so, from the standpoint of disability rights, as well as for many other reasons, it is to be hoped that he never attains the highest office in Germany. However, as a prominent man with a disability who is constantly the object of media attention, he functions as a kind of lightning rod for public debate, whereby those reporting on his politics also create visual images and written texts about disability in Germany today.

The tone and the terms of the debate about whether to include an overt depiction of Franklin D. Roosevelt's disability at the new memorial to him in Washington, D.C. have taken quite different forms. Rather than being an argument over the tactic of aggressive openness in showing and speaking about disability, the controversy here has circled for several years around whether Roosevelt's disability should continue to be concealed in the memorial, given that this was the way he presented himself to the public, or whether new arguments can be made for a sculpture immortalizing him sitting in a wheelchair. Construction of the memorial began in 1990, and at that time the Memorial Commission decided on a sculpture which shows Roosevelt in a typical public pose: sitting on a chair with his long Navy cape draped around him, covering his lower body (frontispiece). The memorial refers to his disability through a time-line inscription noting that after he had polio, he "never again walked unaided," through displaying a replica of the kitchen chair on wheels which he sometimes used, and through the subtle way the statue shows one of his legs to be somewhat withered (which would probably be lost on most viewers). As the chief architect of the memorial, Lawrence Halprin, explained: "Roosevelt was very desirous of keeping his disability out of the limelight. We're not trying to hide it, but it would be going against his desire to evidence it in a sculpture."[37]

As soon as the design of the memorial became public and construction began, disability rights activists and some historians began to protest the omission of a clear depiction of Roosevelt's disability, usually calling for the memorial to include a statue showing him sitting in a wheelchair.[38] From this standpoint, while Roosevelt had correctly done what was necessary more than half a century ago by concealing his disability in order to go on with his career in politics, times had changed. In the years since 1945, the civil rights movement, and specifically efforts of people with disabilities to speak out and act on their own behalf, had begun to lessen the stigma attached to "deviation" from unquestioned "norms." Emphasizing these progressive developments, for example, Rhode Island Secretary of State James Langevin, who has used a wheelchair since 1980, wrote to the Memorial Commission that Roosevelt's decision to conceal his disability was more a testament to his own times, when having a disability was viewed as a weakness, rather than to a "strongly felt personal desire to hide this basic fact about his life from future generations." Langevin, and others criticizing the Commission's decision, went on to suggest that if Roosevelt had been president at a later time, he probably would have been an active force behind the passage of civil rights legislation such as the Americans with Disabilities Act rather than "remaining a silent voice."[39]

As the protests mounted, the Memorial Commission was pressured into releasing a statement on March 1, 1995, addressing issues brought up by those whom it termed "individuals in the handicapped community."[40] This response presented two main justifications for the Commission's refusal to depict Roosevelt in a wheelchair. First, Senator Daniel Inouye, Co-Chair of the Commission, emphasized how important it had been for the U.S. president to present a strong image during the war, stating: "I for one would not want to redo history. FDR was Commander-in-Chief of the greatest fighting force in the world and he wanted to be viewed as a strong leader. I would hate to see the man exploited after he was dead." Second, Curtis Roosevelt, the oldest grandchild of Franklin and Eleanor Roosevelt, gave a more personal justification, recalling his grandfather's stoicism in the face of physical difficulties like this: "He was a very private person and went to great lengths to avoid any discussion or comment on any illness that might be plaguing him." These two perspectives have been echoed in various newspaper columns over the last two years which support the Commission's memorial design.

This point of view considers only the way in which Roosevelt presented himself to the public. It omits, however, any consideration of the reasons why Roosevelt had to choose this strategy, which were rooted in his effort to evade negative stereotypes of disability. Furthermore, it also evidences little consciousness of the ways in which attitudes toward disability have shifted in the intervening years. In its statements, it seems as though it had simply never occurred to the Memorial Commission that issues of disability are important issues of civil rights, and that memorials speak to the present and future, as well as about the past.

As the day for the opening of the memorial approached in the spring of 1997, protests by disability rights organizations against the memorial's design intensified. During one demonstration at the construction site on February 27, for example, I. King Jordan, the first deaf president of Gallaudet University, stated: "If this memorial has no depiction of Roosevelt in a wheelchair, then instead of a memorial to a great American, I honestly believe that it becomes a memorial to hypocrisy."[41] Finally, when disability activists threatened a potentially embarrassing protest at the official dedication of the memorial on May 2, President Clinton agreed to submit legislation to Congress asking that the memorial be modified to include a sculpture clearly depicting Roosevelt in a wheelchair. Supported by sixteen of Roosevelt's grandchildren, as well as by former presidents Bush, Carter, and Ford, Clinton's announcement was welcomed by those who had criticized the Commission's original design.

Roosevelt is a hero to many people with disabilities, and it is thanks to their efforts that the memorial is likely to be modified. However, even the editorials and statements which recently came out in support of showing Roosevelt in a wheelchair generally neglected the larger symbolic importance of clearly depicting his disability, or discussed the importance of such an image only for people with disabilities themselves. The *New York Times*, for example, in an editorial which was certainly well-intentioned, called for modifying the memorial's portrayal of this "inspiring instance of a disability defied and mastered" in order to "give hope and courage to every American similarly burdened."[42] Yet in reality, as Roosevelt knew and many other people with disabilities know today, the "burdens" that we have to face often come less from our particular physical or mental limitations than from the obstacles to living a full life which a biased or insensitive society may place in our way. Seen from this viewpoint, a letter to the editor of the *New York Times* best expressed the meaning of a clear depiction of Roosevelt's disability in this prominent national memorial site: "People with disabilities will be proud to have a statue of Roosevelt in his wheelchair—but it is the nondisabled world that really needs it."[43] For those who continue to view people with disabilities in a patronizing way, such a memorial can highlight the inappropriateness of such pity and condescension. For every employer and for every gatekeeper to our social institutions who have consciously or unconsciously found ways to exclude people with disabilities from full participation, such a memorial can serve as a symbolic witness to the hollowness of their position. And in historical and international terms, such a memorial can also be an important reminder that a man who could not walk was elected to serve as president for longer than any other, and that this man was a leader in defeating fascism, a movement which sought to marginalize and finally eliminate the "unfit" and the "infirm" from the healthy body of the nation.

ACKNOWLEDGEMENTS

I would like to thank the graduate students in the Department of German at Cornell University for inviting me to give a lecture which was my first opportunity to put together the material for this article. I would also like to thank Sander Gilman, Vicki Hill, and Jim Steakley for their encouragement and for providing useful information.

NOTES

[1]Letter to the *New York Times*, April 26, 1997.

[2]"Ein Test für den Kanzler," in *Der Spiegel*, Vol. 45, No. 48 (November 25, 1991), 31. This and all other translations from German are my own.

[3]See Hugh Gallagher, *FDR's Splendid Deception* (New York: Dodd/Mead, 1985) and Betty Winfield, *FDR and the News Media* (Urbana: University of Illinois Press, 1990).

[4]Quoted in Gallagher, *FDR's Splendid Deception*, 63.

[5]On Roosevelt and the National Foundation, see Tony Gould, *A Summer Plague. Polio and its Survivors* (New Haven: Yale University Press, 1995).

[6]Martin Pase (Ernst Pasemann), *Roosevelts Reden und Taten im Scheinwerfer der Presse und der Karikatur* (Berlin: Lühe, 1941). My descriptions of Nazi cartoons are all based on images in this book.

[7]Nicholas Halasz, *Roosevelt through Foreign Eyes* (Princeton: Van Nostrand, 1961), 228.

[8]Pase, *Roosevelts Reden*, 14.

[9]*Ibid.*, 108.

[10]Henry Picker, ed., *Hitlers Tischgespräche im Führerhauptquartier 1941–1942* (Stuttgart: Seewald, 1963), 201.

[11]Obviously, this more "scientific" approach to depicting people with disabilities differs from the Nazis' constant use of antisemitic images. It appears that the Nazis were more reluctant to use negative images of the former group because of fear of alienating the churches or large sectors of the population. And in fact, the Nazis' "euthanasia" program was at least curtailed somewhat due to protests. See "Bishop Galen of Münster protests against euthanasia, August 1941," Jeremy Noakes and Geoffrey Pridham, eds., *Documents on Nazism, 1919–1945* (New York: Viking, 1974), 305–8.

[12]On the propaganda films for sterilization and euthanasia, see Michael Burleigh, *Death and Deliverance. "Euthanasia" in Germany 1900–1945* (New York:

Cambridge University Press, 1994); and Ludwig Rost, *Sterilisation und Euthanasie im Film des "Dritten Reiches"* (Husum: Matthiesen, 1987).

[13]On measures taken by the Nazis against various groups of "deviants," see Michael Burleigh and Wolfgang Wippermann, *The Racial State. Germany 1933–1945* (New York: Cambridge University Press, 1991).

[14]Interestingly, however, the magazine *Stern* imagined at around the same time which politicians it would ideally like to see in the German cabinet, and it published a collaged picture which featured Schäuble as chancellor in his wheelchair in a row with other politicians, integrated into the group (May 14, 1992).

[15]The three cartoons all appeared in *Der Spiegel*, on September 23, 1991, 20; November 25, 1991, 35; and December 16, 1991, 9.

[16]Letter to *Der Spiegel*, December 16, 1991, 9.

[17]See, for example, Philip Reilly, *The Surgical Solution. A History of Involuntary Sterilization in the U.S.* (Baltimore: Johns Hopkins University Press, 1991); and Stefan Kuhl, *The Nazi Connection: Eugenics, American Racism, and German National Socialism* (New York: Oxford University Press, 1994).

[18]According to Reilly, *ibid.*, approximately 60,000 people were sterilized involuntarily under state eugenics laws in the U.S. during a 50-year period ending in the early 1960s. On Germany, see Burleigh, *Death and Deliverance.*

[19]The pamphlet by Karl Binding and Alfred Hoche entitled "Die Freigabe der Vernichtung lebensunwerten Lebens. Ihr Maß und ihre Form" (1920) became one of the main sources for justifications of eliminating "lives unworthy of life" in Germany. See also Rainer Hegselmann and Reinhard Merkel, *Zur Debatte über Euthanasie. Beiträge und Stellungnahmen* (Frankfurt: Suhrkamp, 1991).

[20]The following discussion of the response to Singer in Germany is based largely on his own account: Peter Singer, "On Being Silenced in Germany," *New York Review of Books*, August 15, 1991, 36–42.

[21]See also, Peter Singer and Helga Kuhse, *Should the Baby Live? The Problem of Handicapped Infants* (New York: Oxford University Press, 1985).

[22]See, for example, Franz Christoph, *Tödlicher Zeitgeist. Notwehr gegen Euthanasie* (Cologne: Kiepenheuer und Witsch, 1990). Christoph, who died recently, used a wheelchair as a result of polio, was a prominent disability rights activist in the most radical "cripple scene," and ran for Parliament as a candidate of the Party of Democratic Socialism after reunification.

[23]The best source for following the protests against discussions of bioethics in the disability rights scene in Germany is the magazine *Die Randschau. Zeitschrift für Behindertenpolitik.*

[24]Consider also the fact that Germany is the only country which did not ratify the Bioethics Convention of the Council on Europe, for three reasons: 1) incomplete protection for embryos (in Germany all experimentation on embryos is prohibited), 2) it allows manipulation of the human genome, 3) it allows medical experimentation on persons unable to give their consent under certain conditions. See "Der Streit um das würdige Leben," *Die Zeit*, April 11, 1997.

[25]See Hasso von Henninges, *Arbeitssuchende Schwerbehinderte. Eine Sekundäranalyse amtlicher Statistiken* (Nuremberg: Institut für Arbeitsmarkt- und Berufsforschung der Bundesanstalt für Arbeit, 1993).

[26]On special schools in West Germany, see "Schon als Kind ein geschlagener Mensch," *Der Spiegel*, Nr. 34 (March 24, 1980), 120ff.

[27]Carol Poore, "Disability as Disobedience? An Essay on Germany in the Aftermath of the United Nations Year for People with Disabilities," in *New German Critique*, Nr. 27 (Fall 1982), 161–195. For a recent collection of interviews and

autobiographies of German women with disabilities, see Sigrid Arnade, *Weder Küsse noch Karriere. Erfahrungen behinderter Frauen* (Frankfurt: Fischer, 1992).

[28]See Craig Whitney, "Disabled Germans Fear They'll Be the Next Target," *New York Times,* January 19, 1993; "Germans with Disabilities Fear New Discrimination," Transcript of National Public Radio's "Morning Edition," April 27, 1993; and the documentation of attacks against people with disabilities in *Die Randschau,* Vol. 8, No. 1 (March/April 1993), 17–24.

[29]"Hier herrscht seit '33 Diktatur. Spiegel-Redakteurin Christiane Kohl über den Umgang mit Rechtsradikalen im ostdeutschen Quedlinburg," in *Der Spiegel,* November 9, 1992, 97.

[30]"Knüppel gegen Krüppel," in *Die Zeit,* December 4, 1992, 21.

[31]"Ein Netz und viele Spinnen," in *Die Zeit,* February 18, 1994, 3.

[32]See Oliver Tolmein, "Behinderte raus!?" *Freitag,* Nr. 41 (October 2, 1992), 2.

[33]See Walter Grode, "Behindertenbewegung. Emanzipatorische Perspektiven von Behinderten im wiedervereinigten Deutschland," *Dr. med. Mabuse,* Nr. 74 (October/November 1991), 60.

[34]These blunt depictions of Schäuble contrast with reporting in the U.S. on Max Cleland, the newly elected Democratic senator from Georgia. As a result of being wounded in Vietnam, Cleland had both legs and his right arm amputated. Of course, he is not a candidate for the presidency, but reporting on him is still notable for its restraint in describing his physical condition.

[35]Letter to the editor of *Stern,* Nr. 4 (January 16, 1997), 8–9.

[36]See, for example, the article criticizing Schäuble's politics entitled "Schäuble in seiner reduzierten Fassung," *Die Randschau,* Vol. 7, Nr. 5 (September/October 1992), 5–6.

[37]"Roosevelt's Disability an Issue at Memorial," *New York Times,* April 10, 1995, A10.

[38]Historians supporting a modification of the memorial to show Roosevelt as disabled include Hugh Gallagher, the author of *FDR's Splendid Deception,* and Doris K. Goodwin. The National Council on Disability, an independent federal agency which advises the President and Congress on disability, came out for showing Roosevelt in a wheelchair. The National Organization on Disability was the most active grassroots organization in leading the protests.

[39]Letter of James K. Langevin to Dorann Gunderson, Executive Director of the Franklin Delano Roosevelt Memorial Commission, January 9, 1995.

[40]"FDR Memorial Commission Statement on March 1, 1995 Commission Meeting," 1.

[41]"Disabled Protest Memorial to FDR," *Providence (R. I.) Journal-Bulletin,* February 28, 1997.

[42]"FDR's Last Great Message," *New York Times,* April 23, 1997, A30.

[43]Letter to the editor of the *New York Times,* April 26, 1997.

WILLA SCHNEBERG

PROSTHESIS MAKER

I am not dead.
I guess I'm lucky
to still have one leg
and a job where I can play like the gods
making legs of wood, leather and old tires
for those of us whose karma
is to step on small containers of evil.

I have a lot of time to think
molding calves, kneecaps, ankles, heels.

Because there are so many of us limbless ones,
maybe in two or three generations
mothers will give birth to one-handed
one-legged babies.
Then no one will assume that I am a beggar
built not to be loved.

One night I'll come back to the workshop late
after getting drunk watching the racing boats
at the *Omtuk* Festival to find
that all the pathetic imitations
have become real, brown and fleshy
with splayed toes that will soon know
the goosh of earth and will run
outside and fling themselves
back into the family of the body.

VICTORIA ANN LEWIS

THE DRAMATURGY OF DISABILITY

Disabled characters shaped by the old cautionary and sentimental models of representation have filled the stage for generations, from the stigmatized Oedipus and Richard III to Tiny Tim,
the special child who manifests innocence and goodness in the
world. The success of these depictions can be measured by the
resistance they offer to a new generation of disabled playwrights,
who are attempting to free themselves from those conventions.
The emergence of these new voices would have been inconceiv-
able without the radical change in cultural consciousness
brought about by the disability civil rights movement of the late
1970s. Now after twenty-five years the rag-tag comedy troupes,
the stand-up (or more accurately, sit-down) comics, the agit-prop
collectives, and rowdy performance artists that were the inevitable camp-followers of the political activists and legislators
who changed the social reality of disabled Americans, have
evolved into a new generation of artists. With credentials and
bodies of work that make them competitive with the country's
"best and the brightest," they fearlessly appropriate the narratives of disability as their subject and with skill and imagination
rework the question of identity. This essay will identify some of
the major dramaturgical strategies in this new theater, problems
in reception on both a popular and professional level, and possible directions for future development.

These new voices must always contend with the dominant narrative of disability, a narrative that in the theater, outside of a few
notable exceptions such as *Children of a Lesser God*, has remained
stuck in the past. It is not that the nondisabled theater world
knows nothing about disability and is waiting to be enlightened.
To the contrary, the depiction of disability is over-represented in
dramatic literature. As a result the nondisabled theatrical practi-
tioner often feels he or she knows better than the disabled artist

what is the correct approach to this uncomfortable but irresistible subject—the dramaturgical equivalent of the well-mean-
ing bystander who insists on helping the blind subway traveler by
pulling him or her by the cane toward an unwanted destination.
Rosemarie Garland Thomson describes the intense interest the
nondisabled world has in defining the "deviant" body:

> Corporeal departures from dominant expectations never go
> uninterpreted or unpunished. . . . Cultural dichotomies do
> their evaluative work: this body is inferior and that one is supe-
> rior; this one is beautiful or perfect and that one is grotesque
> or ugly.[1]

We will see that Thomson's "cultural dichotomies" have flourished on the stage and stubbornly refuse to be dislodged. The
old moral and medical models of disability continue to dominate
theatrical depiction, not only because they fill a deep human
need to define ourselves as "normal" against some standard of
abnormality, but also, in terms of theatrical practice, because
they are dramaturgically useful. For example, under the moral
or religious construction of disability, physical difference usually
connotes evil, a punishment for sin, or, to the contrary, desig-
nates beatitude, a blessing from the gods. Consider the ease of
signaling good vs. evil by the addition of a hook, peg-leg, or eye
patch. Introductory guides to screenwriting actually counsel
fledgling authors to give their villain a limp or an amputated
limb. This "twisted body, twisted mind" approach to characteriza-
tion has given us such unforgettable villains as Richard III, Dr.
Strangelove in the Stanley Kubrick movie of the same name, and
Ronald Merrick in Merchant-Ivory's mini-series *The Jewel in the
Crown*. The saint appears as Tiny Tim and Forrest Gump.

The medical model, the historical successor to the moral
model, views disability as an illness. The disabled person is either
charitably removed from society, i.e., institutionalized, or cures
himself, or at least "passes" as cured. The possibility of societal
prejudice and discrimination is never considered in the medical
model. The seductive plot possibilities of the medical model,
with its emphasis on a bodily transformation accomplished by an
isolated effort of will, are irresistible in creating conventional
dramatic structure. Dore Schary's *Sunrise at Campobello*, the 1958
drama based on FDR's efforts to conquer paralysis, paved the
way for the stories of overcoming disability that now outnumber

tales of deformity and monstrosity in the mass media. As Paul K. Longmore notes, the medical model serves as reinforcement for one of the most powerful of all American myths: the rugged individual who pulls himself up by his own bootstraps.[2]

The 1978 play *Whose Life Is It Anyway?* by Brian Clark marks a crossroads in disability depiction. The play and its film adaptation created a furor in the budding disability movement, and movie theaters across the nation were picketed by militant civil rights activists. The play's protagonist Ken Harrison, a quadriplegic due to a car accident, wants to commit suicide after six months in a hospital. As he asserts in his trial, "I'm dead already . . . I cannot accept this condition constitutes life in any real sense."[3] The equation of disability with death, with a life deprived of sexuality or any meaningful work, is diametrically opposed to the message of modern activists and thinkers. But *Whose Life Is It Anyway?* does foreshadow one of the major themes of subsequent disability dramaturgy, the failure and danger of the medical model which deprives disabled persons of autonomy. Arrogant Dr. Emerson is accused of "arbitrary power" and "cruelty" in that he deprives Harrison of choice. What the new generation of writers with disabilities will add to this indictment of the medical model (which is in any case safely sweetened at the play's close) is a construction of disability that places the tragedy of disability not within the individual but within a society that makes participation impossible due to architectural and attitudinal barriers. This social construction of disability, which includes a self-conscious claiming and fostering of community, nourishes the works investigated here and creates new dramaturgical strategies. *Whose Life Is It Anyway?* thus loses its liberal sheen and reveals itself as a convenient celebration of the disabled person who has the decency to alleviate society's collective guilt by eliminating himself.[4]

The simplest way to present the new paradigm of the social model of disability is in stories that directly confront prejudice and discrimination. There is some precedent that such representations can be successful. Retelling the story of sideshow freak Joseph Merrick, the 1979 play *The Elephant Man* by Bernard Pomerance painted an indictment of societal prejudice and exploitation of the physically different.[5] *P.H.*reaks: the Hidden History of Disabled Persons,*[6] developed collaboratively in the Mark Taper Forum's OTHER VOICES Project from 1992–94, at-

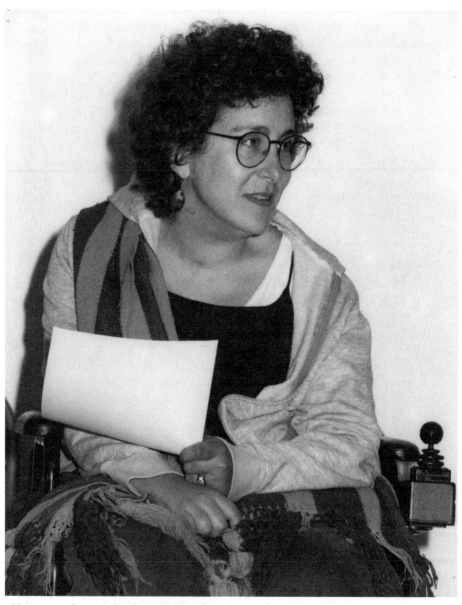

Chicago playwright Susan Nussbaum, author of *Staring Back, The Plucky Spunky Show, Mishuganismo,* and *No One as Nasty.* Photo: Craig Schwartz tempted to introduce the new paradigm of disability by incorporating historical accounts of civil rights actions going back to the thirties and forward to the 1977 takeover of San Francisco Health Education and Welfare Building and beyond. The problem with this kind of storytelling is shared by all "people's theater." How do you create a collective hero? How, as Brecht put it, do you make a five act play about oil? In *P.H.*reaks*, documentary materials such as slides, television coverage, and oral history were interwoven with satirical sketches and naturalistic love scenes. The collective story was balanced with the individual, the political with the personal.

Another emerging strategy is parallel constructions, whether in character or plot, of disability, gender, and race. Young playwright John Belluso, who received an MFA in Playwriting from NYU's Tisch School of the Arts, consciously employs "double and triple identities" in his plays, mixing gender, race, and disability so that the audience has a difficult time reducing the story to the dominant narrative of disability—triumph over tragedy.[7] In Belluso's play *Gretty Good Time*, post-polio Gretty, living in a nursing home in the 1950s and contemplating suicide, first encounters Hiroshima maiden Hideko on the television show *This is Your Life*. Hideko then becomes Gretty's fantasy companion on her journey to escape her "shit body."

Interestingly, the Hiroshima maidens have found their way into a script by Chicago-based actor and playwright Susan Nussbaum. She begins her play *No One As Nasty* by drawing a parallel between her main character, a quadriplegic woman, and the civilian victims of America's first atomic bomb:

> . . . and the Hiroshima maidens got burned and disfigured, there's a word, "disfigured," because of, why? Because—They were in Hiroshima. They were too close to avoid the fire, too far to be consumed. If I was five seconds earlier or later I wouldn't have been hit by a car, my life would be on some different time line, it was an *accident*, it had nothing to do with whether I was a good or a bad person or just an in-between person, we don't live in an ordered universe.[8]

The Hiroshima maidens provide both writers with a potent figure to counter the moral and medical construction of disability. Faced with the horror of the external event of the atom bomb, any interpretation which fixes responsibility for disability on the disabled person becomes obscene.

Other disabled writers have created similar landscapes where race is coupled with physical difference in an effort to demythologize disability. In Mike Ervin's comedy *The History of Bowling*, a disgruntled disabled college student, Chuck, challenges an African-American street preacher who insists that Chuck has brought his disability on himself. Chuck tells the audience:

> And he says to me, "You better get right with Jesus, or he ain't never gonna make you walk!". . . . Who the hell does he think he is? So I turned to him and I said, "You better get right with Jesus, or he ain't never gonna make you white!"

The central conflict in Susan Nussbaum's *No One As Nasty* occurs between a white disabled woman, Janet, and Lois, an African-American personal assistant. As Lois bathes Janet, she ruminates:

> LOIS: At least you belong to a minority where famous stars can suddenly be members and join your movement. It's not like Christopher Reeve is gonna fall off a horse and be black.
> JANET: That's a silver lining. Although I bet Chris sure wishes he could choose, you know? Between being treated with hatred or pity.
> LOIS: Which would you choose?
> JANET: Hatred.
> LOIS: Shows what you know.
> JANET: Yeah, it shows what I know.

By linking disability with race, both playwrights encourage audience members to question the fundamental assumptions with which they approach the disability experience, just as they do with race.

One of the most commonly employed structural reform strategies is the use of more than one disabled character. A solitary disabled figure in a play will inevitably acquire a metaphorical status, and generally that metaphor will reinforce the old paradigms. For example, the "wounded warrior" can serve as manifestation of a wounded or "sick" society in drama ranging from Sophocles' *Philoctetes* to the disabled vet Ron Kovic in *Born on the Fourth of July*. Kovic's impotence in *Born on the Fourth of July* becomes the impotence of a nation engaged in an unjust war against the "feminine" East. Or the reverse valuation occurs: the disabled person becomes a saint, a symbol of all that is good in society. Some recent disabled writing falls into this trap, particularly those narratives focused on celebrating the fact that "Hey, I'm a human being too!" In such a case, the disabled writer, whatever his or her intention, arrives at a personal canonization that leaves the old paradigms of disability intact. The disabled character's personal identity has been rehabilitated, but in the service of the larger cultural myth that privileges personal responsibility over civic or collective responsibility.

To avoid the pull to the stereotype many emerging disabled playwrights create theatrical worlds with multiple disabled characters. *Creeps*, a strong play from the 1970s by disabled Canadian David Freeman,[9] illustrates the advantages of such an approach. Set in a sheltered workshop for men with cerebral palsy, *Creeps* features seven disabled characters with a variety of personality types. This multiplicity makes it difficult to attach the standard brave or bitter mask to the disabled personalities depicted on stage. Similarly, performance artist Cheryl Marie Wade's first full-length, multiple character play, *Gimp Moon*, features three principal roles for persons with disabilities, and several minor ones.

Since the beginning of a conscious disability drama, the most common strategy used to attack received notions of the physically different body has been that of humor. Mikhail Bakhtin, himself disabled, reminds us in his rehabilitation of comedy, *Rabelais and His World*, of the essential relationship between laughter and freedom. Laughter, he tells us, is a "free weapon" to liberate us "not only from external censorship but first of all from the great interior censor; . . . from the fear that developed in man during thousands of years: fear of the sacred, of prohibitions, of the past, of power."[10] Disabled practitioners wielding this "free weapon" of laughter range from the commercial to the radical, but they share a common enemy: "internal and external censors." Back in the 1970s Susan Nussbaum was a student in drama school and acting on the side with a comic street theater company, Rapid Transit, which specialized in issue-oriented "hit and run performances." After a spinal cord injury that resulted in quadriplegia, Nussbaum was recruited for a disabled role in an "inspirational drama" which fortuitously drove her to write:

> It gave me the idea that the wrong way to go was sappy shit, and the right way was shoving our differences in people's faces

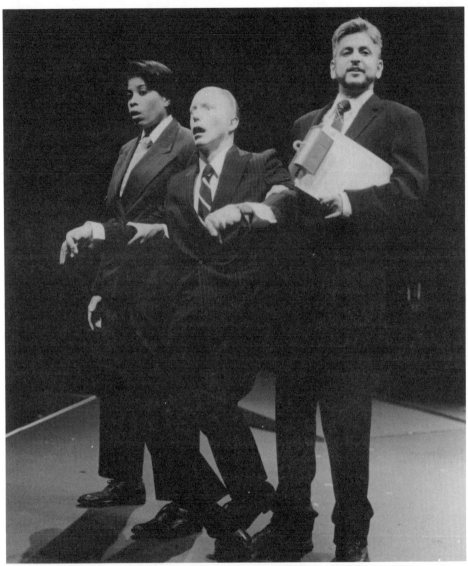

In *P.H.*reaks* two Secret Service officers practice walking an FDR substitute so that in public his disability will be hidden. Photo: Jay Thompson and using humor, the humor in the disability community that had been so much a part of my recovery.[11]

Nussbaum secured a commitment from Chicago's famous improvisational comedy group Second City for the production of a sketch review concerning disability. *Staring Back* was the result, a comedy review using a mixed company of disabled and nondisabled actors that exceeded Nussbaum's expectations: "I was very much surprised at the response. People were standing up every night and screaming." After the success of *Staring Back*, Nussbaum wrote another comedy review with fellow disabled writer Mike Ervin, *The Plucky Spunky Show*, followed by a solo show *Mishuganismo*.

Around the same time that Nussbaum was developing her sketch work, several comedy writers found their way to the OTHER VOICES workshop at the Mark Taper Forum in Los Angeles. First, Nancy Becker Kennedy, whose satirical and musical voice contributed much to the success of OTHER VOICES' two television specials, *Tell Them I'm a Mermaid* and *Who Parks in Those Spaces?* Next, humorists Paul Ryan, Bill Trzeciak, and Vincent Pinto contributed comic sketch material to the OTHER VOICES collaboration, *P.H.*reaks: the Hidden History of People with Disabilities*.

Interestingly, both Ryan for *P.H.*reaks* and Nussbaum for *The Plucky Spunky Show* independently developed scenes with an identical comic premise: a quadriplegic buys some food and tries to eat it and this "courageous" act kicks off a media frenzy. For Ryan it's a hot dog; for Nussbaum it's a container of yogurt. But the point of attack is the same: the perceived incompetence of disabled persons which permits a mundane activity—self-feeding—to be glorified by a self-congratulatory society which can pat itself on the back for being sensitive to the "handicapped" while simultaneously reaffirming its "normalcy."

After reading an account of Franklin Roosevelt's spin control of his disability in Hugh Gallagher's book *FDR's Splendid Deception*, Vincent Pinto found a way to theatricalize this fascinating material for *P.H.*reaks*. In the "FDR" scene two secret service officers practice walking a life-sized dummy, a stand-in for FDR. The older officer explains to the new recruit that their job is to make the public believe Roosevelt can walk because: "He's only as helpless as people think he is." The New Guy is slow to get it:

OLD GUY: You know the president got polio.

NEW GUY: Right. So?

OLD GUY: He *really got polio.*

NEW GUY: So what? He never lets it get him down.

OLD GUY: Well, it got him down more than anyone knows. Crippled him up considerably.

NEW GUY: You're sayin' the President's a *cripple?*

OLD GUY: I'm not sayin' he is a cripple, it just affected his body.[12]

Most of the dramaturgical strategies investigated so far have been aimed at exposing the "constructedness" of the disability identity in order to eliminate it. For example, a society that lionizes a man for eating a hot dog is depicted as mad. Talking about "bitter cripples" is as mistaken as referring to "lazy blacks." A second and somewhat contradictory direction can be observed in these writers—a direction that insists on and celebrates the difference of the disability experience, what is called "disability culture" or "disability cool" in the disability community. Rosemarie Garland Thomson, borrowing from feminist theory, identifies these two tendencies as evidence of a "strategic constructionism" which removes stigma, minimizes difference, attacks hierarchies; and "strategic essentialism" which emphasizes difference and individual experience and calls for a community based on a claimed difference.[13] The two tactics share the common goal of liberating disability from its status as absolute and unchangeable catastrophe.

Very interesting work is emerging from writers that identify primarily with disability culture. Cheryl Marie Wade is one of them. Like many disabled artists, Wade began her theater career late in life. An extraordinarily gifted performer, she rose quickly and deservedly to receive the only solo grant to a disabled artist ever awarded by the National Endowment of the Arts. Wade is pure disabled, born and raised in the disability rights movement, and working-class to her "gnarled" bones. Anyone who has ever heard Wade perform her incantatory poetic-prose will not soon forget it. Recently, declining health has made touring close to impossible for her, so she has turned to conventional dramaturgy, experimenting to see if her unique voice can transfer to a multiple character play. In her work-in-progress, *Gimp Moon,* she tells the story of a disabled activist who kidnaps a baby with a disability as a public relations ploy to alert the public to the dan-

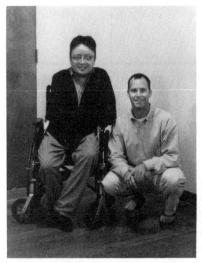 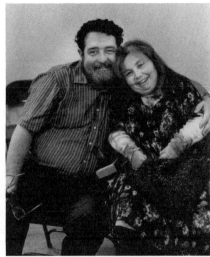

(Left) Playwright John Belluso and associate literary manager for the Mark Taper Forum Pier Carlo Talenti. (Right) Mark Taper Forum literary manager Frank Dwyer and performance artist Cheryl Marie Wade, author of *Gimp Moon*. Photos: Jay Thompson

gers inherent in the right to die movement. Wade asserts that she wants to infuse her play with "the texture of disabled life. I'm creating a crippled world on stage, a world where the *norm* is disability. It's a very real world, but a different one from the majority of the audience."[14]

Susan Nussbaum exhibits a strong essentialist stain and prides herself on including in every piece one joke, one exchange, that is *only* accessible to a disabled audience. Her material is filled with what some in the disabled community affectionately label "crip" humor. Here, for example, from *Mishuganismo*:

> . . . there's a hierarchy of cripdom. There's wheelchair users and there's wheelchair users. As far as most quads are concerned, any crip who has full use of his arms and hands is practically faking it.

Following her own dictum of "shoving our differences in people's faces," all of Nussbaum's writings contain references to disabled lifestyle, details of personal hygiene, such as bathing, dressing, defecating. In fact, a collaborative piece she developed at Remains Theater is titled *Activities of Daily Living*, terminology lifted from Social Security language covering federal assistance to persons with disabilities.

Though Nussbaum definitely allies herself with a disability identity and community, her voice is complex. Equally comfortable talking with disabled vets in Cuba, wrangling in a Marxist study group or sipping martinis at a fictional reincarnation of the Algonquin roundtable, she fashions a complicated dialogue with the disabled and nondisabled audience to create an identity not easily reducible to stereotype. As Rosemarie Garland Thomson says: "Those of us with disabilities are supplicants and minstrels, striving to create valued representations of ourselves in our relations with the nondisabled majority."[15] Or as Nancy Becker Kennedy said in *Tell Them I'm a Mermaid*, "I used to put on the Nancy Fabulous Show. Keep them laughing so they wouldn't feel *so* sorry for me."

But while Susan Nussbaum has been exceptionally well-reviewed by the Chicago press both as a performer and playwright, she has not yet conquered the hurdle erected by the literary departments of the regional, not-for-profit theaters. This is a dubious distinction she shares with another disabled woman playwright, Judith Wolffe, whose writing also tends toward "black comedies."

The "knot" that sets Judith Wolffe's romantic farce *Shelter* in motion isn't a love letter gone awry or the unexpected return of a cuckolded husband, but the complications that arise when post-polio quad Sunny's lover wants to visit her on an off-schedule night. Sunny's personal care assistant can only spare fifteen minutes, time enough to hoist Sunny into bed via a mechanical lift but insufficient for the bathing and hairwashing necessary to prepare for a night of love-making. So Sunny resorts to asking for help from some older women that live down the hall in the rundown project for low-income seniors, where Sunny lives, filling the "handicap" slot required in public housing codes.

Like Wade, Wolffe insists upon the material details of disabled life: transportation snafus, sub-standard housing, underemployment, and erratic personal care. She then inhabits this world with comic characters, the most memorable of whom is Sunny's blue collar, leftist crank of a boyfriend Emmet, who, in his exaggerated despair, envisions "a soup line stretching around the planet." In a tribute to Sunny's endurance, Emmet likens her to the martyred Saint Cecilia. Wild-eyed, he explains: "They cut off her [St. Cecilia's] head, did you know that? Cut it off. Still took her three days to die."[16] The second half of *Shelter* revolves around Emmet's suicidal desires, his wish to take Sunny with him into death, and Sunny's no-nonsense refusal:

> SUNNY: Get serious, Emmet. How many of your friends have died?
> EMMET: A machine shop's a dangerous place.
> SUNNY: Not half as lethal as a hospital.
> EMMET: Working men are killed every day. Boiled to death, crushed, poisoned.
> SUNNY: How many of *your* friends have died? (*Emmet doesn't answer.*) Well, a lot of mine have. You know how I feel? Fuck death. In the ass.

As for Nussbaum, comedy for Wolffe is a matter of life and death. Both these significantly disabled women writers speak from an awareness of their precarious position in a society that has little use for the poor, elderly, or disabled. Furious, on the edge, they use laughter as a weapon to insist on their survival.

Shelter was rejected by the literary department of a southern California regional theater on the basis of the judgment of one reader who felt that Wolffe had "denatured and trivialized" the experience of disability. This dismissal could be seen as a legitimate aesthetic judgment. But several of the writers discussed here have received similar responses to their works in the submission process. Is there a misreading of the emerging works of the disability community? Cheryl Marie Wade observes that most theater professionals "are still looking at *Whose Life Is It Anyway?* as a valid disability play." Is it possible that Wolffe's reader was really looking for a "tragedy to triumph" narrative and perhaps missed the fact that "denaturing" disability was Wolffe's intended effect?

Susan Nussbaum's *No One As Nasty* was rejected by an east coast playwright's organization which found the play, despite its "wit and imagination," to be too "agenda-driven" for their purposes. Even granting the prissiness of the not-for-profit theaters, which consider any passionate political commitment inappropriate for the stage, one would expect a broader dramaturgical response at the close of the 1990s. A host of "agenda-driven" plays—such as George Wolffe's *Colored Museum*, Tony Kushner's

Angels in America, Lisa Loomer's *The Waiting Room*, Robert Schenkken's *The Kentucky Cycle*, and Frank Galati's adaptation of John Steinbeck's *Grapes of Wrath*—have garnered enough Tony Awards, Pulitzer Prizes, box office records and glowing reviews to suggest that the public is not as squeamish as the cultural elite imagines.

John Belluso says,

> It flashes into your head: What might people's reaction be if I wasn't writing about a subject that was so challenging to them? It does seem like another language to many, so set in their seeing disability as an individual narrative and therefore containable. But there's nothing else for me to write about.

Belluso has been criticized for requiring his character Tam in *Traveling Skin* to abandon her wheelchair in favor of crawling, or "slithering," as he puts it. Belluso's response to his critics was, "I wanted to make her movement very slow and painful to the audience, something that will take a lot of time and create unease." In Belluso's desire to discomfort his audience, to disrupt or "alienate" their reading of disability, we can see the influence of Brechtian theory but also perhaps an echo of disability activism. In 1990 at a Washington protest to force the signing of the Americans with Disabilities Act, dozens of members of the most radical arm of the disability rights movement, ADAPT, abandoned their wheelchairs and slowly crawled up the Capitol steps. This action was highly controversial within and outside the disability community. However, ADAPT claims partial victory for the passage of the ADA legislation because of the flood of publicity that followed their collective crawl.

I have a vivid personal memory of a performance which will serve both as a conclusion to this discussion of disability dramaturgy and a hint of a future direction in the field. As the protesting militants reclaimed crawling to make it a noble and beautiful gesture, so did a brief performance at the University of Michigan in the spring of 1995 remind me of the simplicity and possibility of the new representation of the disabled body, not just for those of us who are disabled but for our entire cultural tradition. During the This/Ability Interdisciplinary Conference on Disability and the Arts, actor Brad Rothbart, veteran of the Living Theater and twenty-odd years in a disabled body, strolled down the halls of the University of Michigan's School of Art and

Architecture. Rothbart was naked, his body marked by cerebral palsy, and he carried a small bucket of water. We followed this asymmetrical Pied Piper to an outside courtyard, brilliantly lit by the May sun. Setting down his pail, Rothbart began to bathe himself, sponging water onto his small, tightly-wound body. He traced the outline of his form with the sponge, while his words described a very different body: " . . . squirting soap onto my great left thigh. This leg is thick with muscle. 'Thunder thigh' a lover called it once . . . The Balancer. The Protector."[17] His text was Deborah Abbot's lyrical essay "This Body I Love," in which the speaker celebrates her post-polio body while showering in a public gym. Rothbart continued, "Now to my other. I stroke this slender limb, along the pale sutures whose indelible ribbons mark the times the skin has been incised and peeled open, the bones broken and rearranged. I am tender with this leg. The Small One? The Weak One?" Repeatedly he dipped the sponge into the bucket, bathing his boyish arms and legs, as if he were painting the disabled woman's form onto his own skin.

Rothbart's ritual, with its stillness, its focused simplicity of gesture and voice, interrupted the dominant interpretation and punishment of the nonconforming body, first by presenting the "deviant" body in a fashion traditionally reserved for beautiful female nudes; then by fusing the subject and object of desire in his appropriation of the auto-erotic narrative of a disabled woman; and finally by creating, in his identification with the female "deviant," an enlarged theatrical body capable of extending beyond the personal to the communal and embracing the audience. It was a moment verging on the shamanistic, dispelling deviance, purifying our collective vision. There will be more.

NOTES

[1]Rosemarie Garland Thomson, *Extraordinary Bodies: Figuring Physical Disability in American Culture and Literature* (New York: Columbia University Press, 1997), 8.

[2]Paul K. Longmore, "Screening Stereotypes: Images of Disabled People," in *Social Policy* 16 (Summer 1985), 31–38.

[3]Brian Clark, *Whose Life Is It Anyway?* (New York: Dodd, Mead & Company, 1978), 111.

[4]The most common subject in disability playwriting today, and always from a negative point of view, is the "right to die" issue.

[5]Though this play, like the movie *Mask*, is progressive in that it locates the

problem of disability outside the disabled person, Paul K. Longmore finds both depictions less than salutary. These characters, though more fully characterized than the monsters that preceded them, are incapable of an integrated life in society. Their fate is death.

[6]Doris Baizley and Victoria Lewis, adpt., *"P.H.*reaks*: the Hidden History of People with Disabilities," in Kenny Fries, ed., *Staring Back* (New York: Dutton, 1997). The eccentric spelling of freaks in the title refers to a discriminatory practice of the Works Project Administration(WPA) which stamped a "P.H." for physically handicapped on applications for work by disabled persons and refused all such applicants employment. In 1933 a group of disabled activists, the League of the Physically Handicapped, staged the first known disability civil rights action in America to protest this policy. I am grateful to Paul K. Longmore for sharing his research with us as we developed *P.H.*reaks*. In addition, we studied Robert Bogdan's *Freak Show: Presenting Human Oddities for Amusement and Profit* (Chicago: University of Chicago Press, 1988) for an understanding of the social construction of disabilty.

[7]Interview, October 6, 1997.

[8]Susan Nussbaum, *No One As Nasty*, unpublished, 1996.

[9]David Freeman, *Creeps* (Toronto: University of Toronto Press, 1972).

[10]Mikhail Bakhtin, *Rabelais and his World* (Bloomington: Indiana University Press, 1984), 89.

[11]Interview, October 14, 1997.

[12]Baizley and Lewis, 315–7.

[13]Thomson, 23.

[14]Interview, October 7, 1997.

[15]Thomson, 13.

[16]Judith Wolffe, *Shelter*, unpublished, 1993.

[17]Deborah Abbott, "This Body I Love," in Susan E. Browne, Debra Connors, and Nanci Stern, eds., *With the Power of Each Breath: A Disabled Women's Anthology* (San Francisco: Cleis Press, 1985), 273.

STEPHEN DIXON

THE MOTOR CART

Was it only last week when some guy called and said "Hi, you Mr. Booksomething?" and he said "Yeah, Bookbinder, what can I do for you?" and the man said "Good, I got you. You don't know me but your wife gave me your number and a quarter and said to say she's at Broadway and a hundred-eleventh, north corner of the street on the east side of the avenue, that's what directions she told me to give," and he said "What's wrong, she hurt, spill over?" and the man said "No, but she told me to say her motor cart stopped dead while she was riding it and she can't get it started. I was passing by and she asked would I push her to a phone booth a few feet away, so me and another guy did, but the phone was broken, the whole change part where the coins come down ripped open. And because we couldn't push her to the nearest booth a block away, or she didn't want us to—the cart weighs a ton and she said it was too hot for us to do it, and much as I hate to admit it, she was right—we would have died—she told me to say you should come with the wheelchair so she can get off this hot street and home. So I called you and you know where she's at and you're coming, right?" and he said "One-eleventh, northeast corner," and the man said "I guess it's the northeast—right by the Love drugstore or a few stores away, but downtown from it and that side of Broadway," and he said "Got it. But you're sure she isn't hurt—just the cart that won't operate?" and the man said "Altogether stalled. This guy and me gave it a hefty push to see if we could turn over its engine like a car's after she started it, but it wouldn't because it only runs on batteries, she said, and that she tried every other which way and that she needs the wheelchair. And if you could hurry, she said, that'd be great, and that if I didn't get you would I come back to tell her. But I got you, right?—you're her husband," and he said

109

"Yes, and thanks very much, sir, very kind, for everything," and the man hung up.

Now they're in the country, five hundred miles away, it's sunny and cool, city's still hot they hear on the radio every day and he was glad to get out of it, for another reason because every time she left the apartment something awful seemed to happen to her. He thought after he spoke to the man "What's he going to do now? He can't leave the cart on the sidewalk while he pushes her home in the chair and she can't get home in the chair on her own." The cart he can dismantle, as he's done a couple of times when its lift didn't work and he had to get it into the rear of the van by hand, batteries disconnected and removed, seat taken off and back and pole separated from it, and so on, and he can get the five or six parts into a taxi and carry them to the apartment from the cab and get someone to fix the cart there. But the cart cost more than two thousand and is still in pretty good shape and not insured, so he doesn't want to leave it on the street to be stolen. He can wheel her into an air-conditioned store, he thought, then break down the cart, get it to the apartment and come back for her, unless she has to get home immediately for some reason. But some way, he thought, he hasn't figured it all out yet. Maybe he can drag the cart into a store and say it's worth five bucks to him if they just keep it there for a half hour or so while he wheels his wife home, though he doesn't think any store person would accept money for something like that. Then he went downstairs, wanted to run the four blocks and one long street to where she was but it was very hot and sticky out and he ran about two blocks, stopped because he was breathing so hard, and suddenly sweat burst out of it seemed every part of him and he said "Dummy, what're you doing running in the sun?" and walked quickly in the shade, mopping his head and neck and arms with a handkerchief and when that was soaked, with his T-shirt.

He wants to call his mother today but it's so cool up here and he knows how hot it is in New York, that he doesn't want to hear how bad it is for her. The room she stays in in her apartment is air conditioned and he hopes the air conditioner's working, but she can't get out, she's stuck in that room because of the heat and what it does to her breathing and she knows she'll probably be stuck like that for the next few days, which is how long the radio and newspaper say the heat wave's going to continue there.

When he got to her she was sitting in the cart with her back to him, holding a quarter between her fingertips and looking at the people on the sidewalk coming toward her. "Sally," he said and she turned to him and grinned and said "Oh, wonderful, it's you; I was just looking for someone to phone you. I was beginning to think the man I asked hadn't done it," and he said "No, he got me, was very nice and precise—a good choice: followed your orders to a T-shirt—I only say that because mine's soaked and I want you to know I know it—and repeated your message just the way you gave it, it seemed—Jesus, it's hot. What the hell is it with this weather? Why would anyone ever want to live here, and for the old Dutch, even settle here?" and she said "But he wouldn't even wait till I wrote your name and phone number on a paper. Just said he'd remember and would call you from the next street where he knows another public phone is, and if that one's broken, then the street after that, and took my quarter and flew off." "Well, he did his job; I'd ask him anytime. Now what's the problem, other than the thing not moving?" and got on his knees and checked to see all the wires were connected, and she said "We went through that twice, some men here and I. In fact, one of them who said he's an auto technician, but not of battery-operated vehicles, traced every one of those lines," and he said "It doesn't need new batteries; we got these two last winter and they're supposed to be good for at least two years, and I only recharged them yesterday," and she said "The day before, but I haven't used it much since, so that can't be it." He pulled out one of the battery containers, unplugged and opened it and she said "Wait, where's the wheelchair?" and he looked around and said "Oh my gosh, I didn't bring it. I was in such rush to get here. . . . I'll run back for it," and she said "But what am I going to do in the meantime? I have to pee," and he said "Wait wait wait," and looked inside the container, everything seemed to be in order, closed it and went around to the other side of the cart and unfastened and unplugged and pulled out that container, opened it and saw a nut was loose, the end of some inside wire barely around the battery rod or whatever it's called, and he wrapped the wire tightly around the rod, tightened the nut with his fingers, closed both containers and slid them back onto their platforms and fastened them in and replugged the outside wires and said "You might be moving, don't get startled," set the speed dial to the lowest number, pushed the starter key all the way in and pressed the right side of the driving lever and the cart moved forward a few feet, pressed the left side and it went into reverse, pulled the key halfway out of the starter so the cart wouldn't move. "You did it," she said, "it's working," and he said "Really, I hardly knew what I was doing. Just figured that it was maybe like a lamp that isn't working because of a loose wire, or one that isn't insulated right—the wire, I mean—and is causing some kind of short," and she was beaming and said "It's amazing. Not even the professional auto mechanic could figure it out or even consider that that's what it could be," and he said "He did-n't have the vested interest to look deeper. . . . I bet he didn't even have a vest. Believe me, if it was his own wife—" when a young man said to her "So, you got him," and she said "And he got it working" and put the key all the way in and pressed the lever and the cart moved backward a foot, and the man said "Fantastic, you didn't need your wheelchair," and she said to Gould "This is the gentleman who called you," and the man said "Hiya," and then to them both "Well, see ya," and Gould said "Thanks for calling me; again, that was very kind" and walked be-side her as she drove on the sidewalk toward home, thinking she's got to feel good about what he did, not so much in coming but in figuring out what was wrong and fixing it, when someone tapped his shoulder, it was the young man, who said "Listen, buddy, long as things are working now, I was thinking my call to you's worth a few bucks, don't you think that?" and he said "Jeez, I don't know. . . . I mean, you made a phone call," and she said "I do, give it to him; he went out of his way," and he said "But he was heading that way—weren't you?" to the man and the man said "Sure, but I had to stop, wait for some guy to finish his call; that took me out of the way: in time," and he said "Well, you should be feeling good just that you did something good like that. Why does it always have to be money?" and she said "Please, Gould, stop arguing and do it. He also helped push me to the broken phone with another man, and in this weather, and he would have pushed me to the next corner if I hadn't told him not to," and the man said "The lady's right, I forgot I wanted to do that," and he said "Still, who wouldn't do it for anybody? I'm just saying—" and the man said "Hey, what am I asking for? I go out of my way, work up a fat sweat for her, then ask for a few dol-lars after, and you're holding back when your lady says to give?" and she got her wallet out of her belt bag, Gould put his hand

over it and said "No, I'll do it, don't worry; but I just can't see
why people don't stop and do these things all the time for people who are in trouble, and never with any thoughts of money in
mind," and the man said "I didn't for money. It's something I
only thought of asking for now. And it's fine if you don't need
the cash and do these things, but I'm tight now and a little extra
would help," and he said "Rich, medium income, or poor,
even—everyone, if he or she has the strength, should stop. And
when you don't do it for any kind of remuneration—money and
stuff: a payback, as my dad liked to say—then you know you're
really doing something good," and the man said "Oh screw it,
man," and to Sally "This here what you were about to give?"—she
was holding a five—and Gould said "Not five bucks, that's way
too much," and she said "It would have cost us that much to get
the cart home in a cab," and he said "Yes, but a cabby's got to
charge; a Good Samaritan, though . . . well, one can't be called
that if one's going to ask for money and take," and the man said
"I was what you said then, a 'Good' what you said—I know what
it is. But now, seeing how it all worked out so nice for you, I
thought I could use the money and you'd feel good in giving it
because of the way it went," and Gould said "Boy, does he have a
line. Anyway, I give up," and walked away and stopped, his back
to them, and thought she's probably giving the guy the five; or
maybe he's now saying "Actually, if you have a ten that'd be even
better," and she'd give that too. She gives and gives. Whatever
charity or institution or organization sends her an envelope
through the mail asking for a donation, for this or that cause except for some blatantly crazy or politically antipathetic one, she
writes out a check. "What's three dollars?" she's said, or "four" or
"five," and he's said "Not worth the time to write out the check
and for them to cash it. But they put you on their sucker list and
other charities and do-gooding and -badding organizations buy
those lists and every other month send you requests for dough
and you give three to five bucks to them without checking if
they're legit or if ninety percent of the money they collect goes
to soliciting that dough. And you also get on those groups' lists
and they're sold, and so on and so on, till we end up getting six
to seven solicitations a day through the mail or over the phone
and some so preposterously unethical in the way they ask for
money—'urgent' it'll say on what looks like an authentic express
letter when it's actually been sent bulk rate—that they ought to

be reported to the attorney general of the state," and she's said "Now you're exaggerating," and he's said "Maybe, but only by a little," or "Hardly—I've barely touched the tip of the ice pick." She pulled up to him right after the incident with the man and said "Now that was unnecessary," and he said "I'll clue you in as to what was unnecessary," and she said "Listen, sweetie, he helped me when I needed help the most, and that counts for something," and he said "He weaseled five to ten bucks out of you for what should have been . . . well, I already said too much about what it should have been for: the good feeling he was supposed to get," and she said "It could be he not only feels good now that he helped me but also feels a few measly dollars richer. So what's wrong with that if you're hard up for cash?" and he said "Ah, you schmuck, you know nothing," and she said "What!" and he said "Sorry," and she said "No you're not; screw you too, you bastard," and rode off and he walked after her and when she turned the corner at their street he thought "Oh, the hell with her," and ducked into the bookstore there to look through the literary magazines and he wasn't in there a minute, holding a new magazine he hadn't known of but which looked good because of the artwork on its cover, when he thought "Will she make it all right into the elevator? She can do it by herself most times, but sometimes the cart gets stuck, especially when she backs out of the cart into their hallway, and if she has to pee badly she can get flustered opening the apartment door and working the cart into the foyer," and put the magazine back and left the store and ran down the block and caught up with her at the elevator and the moment he stopped, sweat burst out of him again, even from his legs this time it seemed, and he stood beside her, wiping his face with his wet handkerchief and then with the bottom of his wet shirt, till the elevator came and she drove the cart inside it while he kept his hand over the slot the door comes out of, then he got in and pressed their floor button and they rode up silently, she staring at the wall she faced.

SANDRA M. GILBERT

E-MAIL TO THE DEAD

In 1991, when my husband quite unexpectedly and shockingly died following routine surgery, he had been banking electronically for six or seven years, although neither he nor anyone else we knew "did e-mail," as the saying goes.

Elliot paid bills in the garage we'd long ago converted into a study for him, using a clunky old Kaypro whose CPM operating system was even then obsolete, although it's still perfectly workable. The machine was, I think, one of the first to come with an internal modem, which my husband attached to a phone line that he'd moved so it emerged rather oddly from the floor, as if it were an umbilical cord enigmatically linking him with a host of buried accountants. Sometimes when I picked up the phone in my own study (inside the house), I could hear the cadenza of tones, hasty and decisive, that said his computer was dialing the Bank of America. More often, my receiver was clogged with the high-pitched wail that means somebody is on line.

Nevertheless, I understood little about what he was doing, even though I would often boast at parties about his mystifying prowess at homebanking. And I understood still less but was even more impressed when a year or two before he died he learned how to access our campus library's on-line catalog and was actually able to print out useful lists of reference books for both of us.

Yet though I believed he knew such a lot about what to do with a modem, Elliot died before he could really grasp the nature of the tools he was using, much less their implications. He'd heard of e-mail, for example, but assumed he'd have to be in his office to "do" it, not realizing that for the price of a local call the same clunky home computer he used to reach his bank could telnet him to our university and thence around the world.

Of course, his ignorance (and mine) hardly mattered at that

115

point, some seven years ago, because only the most advanced and eccentric of our colleagues had the slightest interest in the mode of weirdly disembodied communication called "e-mail." Indeed, even the notion of faxing seemed remarkably twenty-first century and sci-fi to most of us. My husband was then the chair of the department where I still teach, and I remember trying without much success to persuade him that he ought to ask the dean for funds to buy a facsimile machine for the office. His administrative assistant advised that this was an extravagant request, he told me firmly. How could he have imagined that within a year or two of his death such equipment would be considered not only a *sine qua non* but a rather old-fashioned one in most academic departments?

Lately it's occurred to me that as a way of thinking grief has much in common with speculative fiction. Both, after all, are about alternative lives—past, present, or future. *What if,* cries the griever, just as the sci-fi writer does. *What if* the calamity hadn't happened, the survivor broods, *what if* the dead one I loved were still alive? What would my life be like today? How would *he* be living—and how would I? And the writer of speculative fantasy asks similar questions. Two or three decades ago, for example, storytellers publishing in *Fantasy and Science Fiction*—the most famous and popular magazine of its kind when I was growing up—might have wondered *What if* the sentences we have for centuries inscribed on stacks of recycled forest fiber should dematerialize and whiz off around the globe at almost the speed of light?

Along with the sci-fi writer, the fantasist, and the teller of ghost stories, the griever is always on the edge of another universe, a cosmos that aches with possibility like a phantom limb.

What if the surgeon's knife hadn't slipped (as it very likely did), I ask myself on the most perilously speculative days, *what if* the residents had been more competent, *what if* the nurses had been more watchful, *what if* my husband had lived with me through these seven long years that have followed his disastrous operation?

As everyone who has grieved knows all too well, the answers to such questions come in countless forms, some tediously general and some almost bizarrely particular. *If* the surgeon's knife hadn't slipped, I sometimes tell myself, I would have slept well at night, hence awakening peppy and refreshed, for most of the last seven years, which is no doubt a true but also a quite uninteresting point. *If* the residents had been competent, I muse, I would have spent lots more productive time in the seaside house where my husband and I loved to go together to work—another not terribly fascinating idea.

If Elliot had survived the surgery, he would now have an e-mail address. I regard that as one of my better insights.

Everyone in my department now has an e-mail address. Mine is sgilbert@ucdavis.edu. My husband's would be elgilbert@uc-davis.edu. And just the way, for the sheer fun of it I sometimes thought, Elliot used to log onto his homebanking system too often, with a clatter and scuttle of life across the keyboard of the Kaypro, he'd now log on to his e-mail three or four times a day, inscribing a newer, faster computer with his user name—"el-gilbert"—and a secret password whose contours will alas always have to stay secret.

(Would it be "Kipling" or "Dickens," in honor of authors whose works he studied? Would it be, like his ATM password, our two sets of initials put together—"elg" and "sem"—to celebrate our marriage? Would it be his birthday or mine or maybe our grandson Val's? I can't know it, I'll never know it, but I can virtually see the rapid two-finger technique, the virtuoso brio and panache, with which he'd deliver that magic word into cyber-space.)

I can *virtually* see: the alternative universe the dead inhabit, the hypothetical cosmos in which we who are bereaved live out the lives we would have or might have or should have had *if* the chance of grief had not been dealt to us—when I'm most be-mused I feel as though that cryptic space is itself eerily compara-ble to the virtual realm into whose unseen folds we aim our daily e-mail.

Grief constructs invisible interlocutors, absent presences who read the stories we send into air, into thinnest air, and who are our cherished companions in the imaginary rooms of what might have been. Ever since the catastrophic day when my hus-band's life was inexplicably severed from mine, I've talked to him "in my head," as we mourners often put it. But lately, since I realized he'd have an e-mail address by now, I sometimes find myself standing before the glittering screen of the night sky and posting messages toward the virtual place where I wish he'd be waiting to read them.

Dear E., I might say, *I just got back yesterday from a trip to Ithaca, where I went to Val's karate class. He's eleven now, remember? And just got his purple belt. Let's think about how to celebrate. But in the meantime, there's a dept. meeting tomorrow where we're going to discuss X's promotion, and I'm just not sure what to think about the case as it's been presented to us. Could you please write back with advice asap? Lots of love and xxx xxx xxx forever, sem.*

Of course, I couldn't send this message to what would have been my husband's e-mail address had he lived. It would have to go to a different, more appropriate and accurately specified "place," wouldn't it? In my upbeat moments, I imagine this "real" virtual address as "elgilbert@cosmos.mys," a textual string in which, just as in ordinary e-mail "edu" stands for "educational" and "com" for "commercial," "mys" stands for "mysterious."

ELI CLARE

TO THE CURIOUS PEOPLE
WHO ASK, "WHAT DO
YOUR TREMORS FEEL LIKE?"

Tell me: have you ever watched
hands play a piano? Fingers
on the keys, ivory to skin, dance
white to black and back again, run
wild and loose, thump and caress
the universe cradled inside
a baby grand, those hands I lost at birth.
Breath strangled to nothing,
like falling I came into the world,
brain of my fingers half dead.
Explain to me your hands resting
still as water before they dance.
That I cannot imagine.

REGINALD SHEPHERD

ABOUT A BOY

Everything derives from wreckage, returns
there soon enough. He is what sees and hears
when no one's here, the self assembled
as disguise, grayscale paradox, this paradise

of stone. He's heat behind glass, these days
marred by his various collisions
with perfection. Outside him there's light
captivated by the mumble of summer wind

through heavy branches stumbling under green,
there's the impercipience of men's useless bodies
striding past blind trees, but there's no safety
there. This song that won't go out of them,

their bodies never hear. That sky's retracting
its threat of rain, where lack is a rebel bird again,
starling or any interloper laughing
through the air we breathe, others'

air as well. His skin breathes centuries of dust
and other residues, as if it never
had been damaged, his almost
unforgivable youth has hardened,

and will not be moved. How moving
his remains become, how helpless
under glass. Never doing the things he wants
to the bodies he wants to do them

to. Poor Eros. His arms are broken off
at the shoulder, his eyes have worn
shut. How can he shoot vagrant birds
from his sky? He can't remember

things: that men are not statues
after all, that time is a traitor whispering
as you desire me, and other lying items
of this world: a moment's shimmer

of summer leaves, this shaft of noon caressing
a stone nipple in passing. Things marble learns
to say, but silently. He doesn't know the nothing
he is when he's not known (vanished landscape

of skin), isn't himself from time
to time. Eros is bitter, and bitterly proud.

DALLAS WIEBE

THE THIEF

I'm a forgetful man. I forget everything. Sometimes I forget my telephone number, my address and my age which, I think, is seventy-five. I've been forgetful for as long as I can remember, which isn't very long. If I remember correctly, I was forgetful as a child. I was told by my parents, whoever they were, that when I went to kindergarten for the first day I told the teacher my name was Frank. That wasn't correct, of course. Maybe that wasn't the name I used. I don't know anymore. Someone might explain to me what is meant by "kindergarten." Later on, if I can remember what my real name is I'll tell you. Maybe I'll remember my address and my phone number so that you can write a letter or call me and remind me who I am. My doctor, what's his name, says I might be developing Alzheimer's disease. He says I'm the right age for it. Luckily, I can't remember my age or what that disease is so I don't know what he's talking about.

Because of my forgetfulness I lose things. Sometimes I even lose myself. I walk out the door and forget why I went outside. I wander around and wonder where my door is. I know I'll recognize it if I see it. My wife Vera sometimes comes out and leads me back. She wants to put a sign around my neck: "Point this mumbling wreck back to 75 East Pomeroy. He's harmless." I forget to put on the sign most of the time and I'm not sure that's my correct address anyway. When I do put the sign on I can't remember what it's for. I stay in our house most of the time but I'm not sure why. I stay in the house and wonder who I am.

My wife Priscilla once decided to get me into some religious activity in order to help my memory. She took me to a church that was Methodist, Presbyterian, Episcopalian, Roman Catholic, or Christian Science. One of those anyway. But it didn't work. I couldn't remember whether fishes were turned into loaves or loaves into fishes. I couldn't remember whether there were three, four, or eight Disciples. I couldn't remember the difference between Jesus of Nazareth, Jesus Christ, Christ Jesus, the Savior, or the Messiah. They all sounded the same to me. I got confused about who was crucified and who did the crucifying. I couldn't remember if the Nazarene was hung right side up or upside down. I was never sure who arose from the dead and who stayed dead. I didn't know whether to chew the wine or drink the bread.

When religion didn't work, my wife Marilyn got me a pet. It was a dog, a cat, a rabbit, or a mouse. I'm not sure which. It might have been a hamster. Anyway, it had fur on it and it ran around. I named it Kathy, Mary, Geraldine, Harold, or Jack, something that too has faded away. I tried to teach the pet, whatever it was or whatever it was called, to sit up and beg, to speak, to bring me my newspaper, and to play dead. That didn't work because the pet was always under a table, a chair, or a cabinet. The one thing I do remember is that when I took the pet for a walk it always seemed to know the way home. The pet died, ran away, or my wife Genevieve gave it to a neighborhood kid. The smell remained in the house, but because all pets smell the same that didn't help my memory either.

Not knowing who I am doesn't bother me. Not having a religion or a pet doesn't bother me. It's losing things that gets me worried. Often I lose them right on the table in front of me. That's what I thought was happening when I began losing books. I'd put a book down on a table, walk away and come back and the book would be gone. My wife, whose name is Ariadne, Portia, or Celestina, or whatever, said, "Melvin, you are just being forgetful as usual." But after losing several books, I decided to go on the offensive. Or is it the defensive? I figured out how to fool my wife, my doctor, and the thief. I started writing down what I left and where I left certain items, especially my books. That's how I came to know that the books were being stolen. When I realized that, I decided on another step to help my memory. I decided to structure the thievery. I decided not to be a victim of my own failing and the arrogance of the thief. I decided to make a list of things to be stolen. I decided to educate the thief. I decided to select the best titles for him.

The first book I deliberately put out on the library table for the thief was one of my favorites: *Mysticism in the Republican Party* by Elizabeth Glimmer. At least, I think that's what it was; I seem to have lost my notes. The book disappeared. The next book I put out was, I think, *Can the Dead Feel the Cold?* by Ernest Calvin. It disappeared. I'm fairly certain that the third book I put out was *Werewolves and Self-Esteem* by Tony Trasha. It was gone in the morning. I know in my heart that the fourth book I put out on the table was Pierre Crozier's *The Right Cross: A Life of Jesus.* It was gone before I finished writing down the title and where I left it. The fifth was *The Memoirs of Judas Iscariot* by Thomas Rotbaum. The sixth: *Prestidigitation in the Eucharist* by Willy Faust. Then came, I think, *The Tattooed Trunk* by Burney Nagle, *Empowering the Shakers* by Felix Trembly, Phyllis Rantly's *Marxism and Greed* and her second book *Marxism in Georgia,* Jill Scentley's *Death in the Kennel, Bulging Guts and Rubbery Butts* by Victoria Pillow, Bob Mariner's *Philosophy in the Flophouse,* and Jim Callous's *Armageddon and After: The Life of Dan Quayle.* If my memory serves me correctly, the last book I put out was my all-time favorite: *The Love Life of Emily Dickinson* by Jerry Stones. All disappeared.

I think I thought for a moment that I had truly lost the best of my library. I think I thought that I had not fooled the thief. He had fooled me. But then you know what happened? A miracle. The books started coming back. And they came back annotated. I paged through *The Love Life of Emily Dickinson,* the first book to come back onto my library table, and found on page seventy-five, "Lust and poetry have nothing to do with each other. Sex is forgotten before it happens." *Armageddon and After* came back the next night. On page sixty-four the thief had written, "The four last things are a motel, divorce, re-marriage, and Indianapolis, Indiana." *Philosophy in the Flophouse* came back with, on page fifty-five, "Memory is the virus of time. It weakens the body until it succumbs to its own self-generated disease. Forget it." *Bulging Guts and Rubbery Butts,* page forty-nine, "The universe is infinitely expandable. The expansion cannot be girdled by the human mind. Hot air cannot be contained." *Death in the Kennel,* page forty-three, "Every day is a dog's day. Pets are the guarantee of our immortality. Sweet pooch, I love you." *Marxism and Greed* and *Marxism in Georgia* came back together. In the first book, on page forty-two, "Who was Karl Marx?" and in the second on page forty-one, "Who cares?" *Empowering the Shakers* said, page forty, "'Tis the gift to remember; 'Tis the gift to forget. You bet." *The Tattooed Trunk,* page thirty-nine, something I didn't understand: "The mind trembles at the bark of the elm. The runes of limbs compose the vestiges of inertia." *Prestidigitation in the Eucharist* said, page thirty-eight, "The right hand is the flesh; the left hand is the blood. Shake hands and you do something in remembrance of someone." *The Memoirs of Judas Iscariot*, page thirty-seven, "Never trust paper money." *The Right Cross: A Life of Jesus*, page thirty-six, "Never trust shepherds and wisemen. Be a carpenter. Join the union." *Werewolves and Self-Esteem*, page thirty-five, "The Moon has nothing to do with the mind of man. Darkness comes in howling and egotism." *Can the Dead Feel the Cold?*, page thirty-four, "Only in the sense that the mind goes blank. Death and coldness are easily forgotten ideas." Finally, *Mysticism in the Republican Party* came back blank. I guess there was nothing for the thief to say. He probably just trembled at the verge of perception.

I'm pleased that the thief was an honorable person. Whoever he was I thank him for returning the books and for sharing his thoughts with me. I'll forget them soon, but, for now, they linger on the edge of oblivion. I recall now the books I put out for the thief. The first one was *Mysticism in the Republican Party*. The last one was *The Love Life of Emily Dickinson*. My memory is improving. I know I can be just as filled with memories as the next person. I know I can forget just as easily as the next person. I remember thinking, once, that, given what I am and in order to serve mankind, I could be a kind of repository of things not worth remembering. Just think of what an archive that would be. It would erase the mind. Perhaps that's where I started forgetting everything. No one should ask himself what is worth remembering. The answer is obvious.

For some reason, I remember now what it was like when the last of the books was stolen and before any were returned. I remember how comfortable it was when my library table was empty. There was nothing to read, nothing to think about and nothing to bother the tranquillity of emptiness. I think that's it. Emptiness is what it's all about. There's something to be said for losing it all. To experience nothing, to sit in oblivion, to have the mind at a dead stop, that's for me. To experience nothing, the idea of nothing, the presence of nothing, that's for me. To be completely anonymous, unidentifiable, unrecognizable even to oneself, that's what it all comes down to.

I am a bit confused though. My books are back with their annotations but my wife Polly says the books never left my library table. I can't remember what she's talking about. She says the notes are all in my handwriting. I can't be sure about that because I can't remember what my handwriting looks like. She says, "Chris, you wrote those notes. I saw you do it." When I asked her why she called me "Chris," she said that my name is Christian Freund and that I'm seventy-five years old. Perhaps someone will write me or call me to let me know if she's telling the truth. Otherwise I guess I'll know if she's telling the truth about my name and my age if I can find my birth certificate. I know I have one. I'm just not sure where it is.

MARK DEFOE

AT WALDEN'S IN AUGUSTA MALL,
WE MEET THE READER
COME DOWN FROM THE MOUNTAINS

Out of some hollow, the woods colt,
archetype, spawn of foul coupling,
child-man with a sister mother,
escapee from our closed album.
He comes to gibber, to remind
us that he is our kin. He barks
at the comix, poking a lean
finger at Batman and Robin,
babbling goofiness to Goofy.
Toothless and grizzled, one foot east,
one foot west, he yelps as if he
has found his long lost friends, as if
this rack of cartoon characters
had been his chapter and his verse.

Readers peek from concordances,
blend into their erudition,
dive deep into glossaries.
Is he harmless? Is that English?
God, that sounds like cousin Clevis.

Escorted out, waddling like Chaplin,
he who-whos the teeming hallway
like Daffy Duck. A young clerk says
he gets loose from his Aunt Neva
when she comes for her speed walking.
He speaks in tongues; enroll him
in your reader's club, I suggest.

She is not amused. Suddenly,
my words seem walls. Ashamed, I flee.

His staccato oratory
echoes in my skull—mad reader,
calling from that time when forest
stretched hill beyond hill, yarping a
lingo savage and strange, shrill with
something like longing, something like joy.

BROOKE HORVATH

READING *THE GINGERBREAD MAN* WITH MY DAUGHTER

Read, read, as fast as you can
is what I want to say but don't,
for that is what she is already doing
though moving painfully slowly
from word to word as through
something viscous as first
the old woman, then the children,
the horse, the cow, the cat
try to catch the Gingerbread Man.

She is at times a better guesser
than reader, trying
after a peek at the picture
to slip "stove" past me
where the word is "oven."
When I point to ask if that's
the word for "stove,"
she snuggles closer, grins,
says, "Daddy, I believe so."

Sitting on the porch,
we puzzle over morphemes
like two Talmudic scholars,
our reading as labored
as any fundamentalist's,
so tedious I wonder how
she can be following the plot,
its cookie-against-the-world
conflict, its paranoid's vision

of enemies everywhere,
its message of inevitable defeat,
of the brief ripple loss
leaves in its wake,
of indifference to how
the different suffer.
But she croons each "Stop! Stop!"
knowingly, like a seduction,
shouts melodramatically
the hero's brash refusals,
laughs at each escape.

She, too, right now,
would like to get away from me,
but tomorrow must deliver to her class
a report about this horrible story
she has been assigned,
and already, seven weeks
into this new school year,
her teacher, who knows
only one way to teach,
and the principal,
who has said he wants no
"special needs" kids in his school,
have given up on her,
are looking for excuses
to get rid of her.

And so we'll stay here, the book
between us, until the light fails
or we have finished,
although each time anyone
passes on the street,
she must pause to say hello,
to wave and wait for a reply,
which most of the time she gets.
When not, she squints, watching
some jogger or dog-walker pass,
her face screwed up expectantly,
her lips whispering
"hello?   hello?   hello?"

until I recall her to our task,
encourage her to read more quickly,
enunciate more clearly,
as though by speeding through this book
she might outrun her fate,
as though a good report
will change the principal's doughy
smile into something real,
as though knowing which letters
spell "oven" will make true
her teacher's smiling lies
about the school doing all it can.

And so I urge her on
past another foe, the dog
this time, until a clique
of school friends bicycles by
and she must rush to the curb
to call hello. I try
to coax her back, shout
that we've just a few pages left,
but she knows how this story ends,
knows all about the fox
on the last page
who will eat the Gingerbread Man
because after all that is exactly
what gingerbread men are made for.

I yell, "Stop! Stop!"
imitating her, imitating
the old woman, the children,
the horse, the cat, the cow,
her teacher, her principal,
wanting to chase and catch her
so we both can run as fast as we can
and cry to everyone we pass,
that they can't catch us.

But I sit, watching the girls
pass by. Each smiles and waves,
but no one stops,

and my daughter stands
a moment longer, arm up,
eyes following, hand moving
in a gesture of greeting
and farewell.

ANNE RUGGLES GERE
CYNTHIA MARGARET GERE

LIVING WITH
FETAL ALCOHOL SYNDROME/
FETAL ALCOHOL EFFECT (FAS/FAE)

Even the title of this essay raises uncertainties. How shall we call this disability that shapes our lives? The medical model, which inscribes much of disability's discourse, draws on a dynamic body of research, and terms keep changing. In 1973 Fetal Alcohol Syndrome (FAS) was the term used to describe the neurological and physical consequences of pregnant mothers drinking alcohol. In 1978 medical researchers introduced the term Fetal Alcohol Effect to describe persons who did not have all the physical or neurological markers characteristic of Fetal Alcohol Syndrome. In the past year or so the term Alcohol-Related Neurodevelopmental Disorder (ARND) has been proposed, but many clinicians criticize its vagueness and recommend the more comprehensive term (FAS/FAE).[1] Because it is the most commonly used, if not most precise, term, we use FAS/FAE, but over the years Cindy and I have described her condition as FAS or FAE as well as FAS/FAE.

It is not news to say that most representations of disability have been constructed by those outside the bodies of the disabled. Doctors, social workers, therapists, and researchers provide much of the language we use to talk about disability. A few accounts of disability are inscribed by the disabled themselves, but these, to the extent that they rely on verbal language, are shaped by terms drawn from discourses of pathology. In addition, such narratives tend to focus on the individual author, giving relatively little attention to the social dimensions of disability. In this essay we underscore the human relationships that surround disability by combining our two voices and calling on the alterna-

133

tive language of images to represent our related experiences of living with and inside Cindy's body.

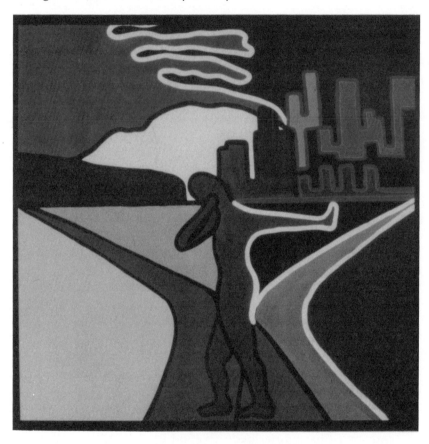

There are many names that describe who I am, and each has its own place. I am from the Athabascan people who live as far north as the Brooks Range, east to Hudson's Bay, west to the Kuskokwim Mountains, and my Navaho and Apache cousins live near the Grand Canyon. My nation is Dene, the people. I am a Kaska, of the Nehoni or Wolf people. My band is the Liard River Band. This is where the trap line of my grandparents, Mike and Magdelan Johnny, runs. On my mother's side is the Kaska, and on my father's the Tahltan. In the traditional way, I follow my mother's clan. As a Wolf Clan woman I follow the rhythms of the land and the way of the elders. The pride of my nation runs as deep as my blood within me.

One of my names is Kulimā, given to me by my grandmother Magdelan, who is still alive and up in her nineties. This sacred blood name comes from my grandmother's grandmother. In the white world I carry two names. One is Cindy Ann Johnny, and the other is Cynthia Margaret Gere. I received the first when I was born and the second when I was adopted. Cynthia Margaret Gere is my legal name, but those who know me best call me Woman of the King Salmon. This last name I carry with pride because the King Salmon fight their way up the Yukon River and the Ross River in Kaska country to spawn. I choose the way of my Athabascan ancestors.

When Cindy joined our family at age three and a half, she was a very active child. "Please use your words," her father Budge and I would beg when she stuck her fingers into the middle of a just-frosted cake, grabbed a stuffed animal from another child, chased the dog round and round the coffee table, or stuffed the Montessori school's paste into her mouth. She quickly earned the nickname "Zoomer." Because she was our first child, we had few expectations about her development; because we were her fourth family, we assumed she would need extra time to grow. Cindy's lively interest in the world and her outgoing nature convinced us that she would soon catch up. When she couldn't name "red," "blue," or "green" we checked for color-blindness, but difficulties tying her shoes, learning to distinguish right from left, and telling time seemed reasonable for a child who had experienced so many changes in her short life. I marveled at her creative phrases like "cloth paint" (for printed fabric) or "blue sky day" (for sunny day), but I noticed that she often referred to classmates as "my friend" because she couldn't recall the name and used circumlocutions like "when we have toast and cereal in the morning" because she couldn't retrieve "breakfast."

After a second year of kindergarten Cindy was classified as "ready" to read, and two years later her teacher wrote that she had "been introduced to all beginning and ending consonants and short vowel sounds," but still had "difficulty seeing words as whole units." Budge and I began to wonder whether Cindy needed more than time and, at the urging of her teachers, agreed to have her tested. The psychologist advised us to accept the fact that Cindy would have difficulty graduating from high school and certainly would not be college material. Attempting to encourage us, she wrote, "It may well be that one will be able to consider the mainstreaming of this young girl into traditional education programs in several years."

Across fourteen years of schooling (in addition to repeating kindergarten, Cindy took an extra year in elementary school) we tangled, pleaded, and strategized with teachers and schools, trying to create situations where Cindy could learn and at the same time keep her self-esteem. She spent two years in Montessori school; three in a public primary school known for its affirmation of diversity; three more in a private school for learning-disabled students; two in a public intermediate school where a good friend served as principal; and four years in three different private middle and high schools. Finally, she spent her junior and senior years in a public high school that provided a vocational program in visual merchandising as well as resource room support for students with learning disabilities. Kay, one of the special educators in the resource room, met with teachers to discuss Cindy's assignments, help with homework, and demonstrate ways of organizing time and work. Best of all, she persuaded the principal that the graduation requirement in math could be met by taking an untimed test with a calculator and then worked with Cindy for days and days to complete it. She became, in her own words, "Cindy's mom at school."

Our family began each school year full of hope. In September of 1981, for example, I watched Cindy straighten her new blue skirt around her pencil-thin waist, helped her with the stiff buckles on her new shoes, and French braided her long dark hair. We were both excited because she was starting at a new school. I clung to the hope that maybe this time we'd found the place where Cindy could start learning, that maybe this year she would begin to read confidently. At age twelve she would be entering the fifth grade. She expressed some self-consciousness about being older than the others in her class, but her delight at being able to ride the bus with the neighborhood kids soon triumphed. Her eyes shone as she picked up her lunch box, and she stood tall as she walked to the corner bus stop. I was so excited I organized a neighborhood potluck to celebrate the first day of school. Three weeks later my heart ached as I helped Cindy buckle her scuffed shoes. A wrinkle of concern had appeared between her eyes, and she hung her head as she shuffled out the door. It was Friday and despite hours of flash cards and singing games she still couldn't spell the ten words that had been assigned on Monday. Her classmates were working on multiplication while she struggled with adding and subtracting single digit numbers. The report from the remedial reading teacher said she had trouble decoding two-syllable words.

I never expected to attend my daughter's college graduation, but on May 12, 1996, I stood outside the gymnasium at the University of Alaska at Fairbanks enjoying the view of the Alaska Range and watching the graduates step out of the line of mortar boards for one more picture. Cindy, dressed in her traditional regalia of buckskin dress and Athabascan-style beaded moccasins, stood out in the sea of black. She and four or five other graduates chose to wear Native clothing, rather than Geneva gowns and mortar boards, to express pride in their traditional culture. Inside, when the dean's voice intoned, Cynthia Margaret Gere, Bachelor of Fine Arts, I recalled the teachers who wrote "Cindy excels in creative activities," "she draws with impressive flair and imagination," and "shows real talent in art." They confirmed what I knew since the day I watched a tiny Cindy, frustrated by my lame attempts at Halloween decorations, cut, freehand, witches, cats and broomsticks with her rounded kindergarten scissors: Cindy is an artist. Seeing Cindy's senior thesis show, "On Deaf Ears: An Athabascan Perspective," confirmed this truth once again.

When I walked into the gallery I was overwhelmed by the overall effect of large (4'×4') paintings intermingled with carvings and leather work Cindy had produced in her Native Arts courses. Then I heard one of the art professors say, "This is one of the strongest shows I've seen in this gallery," and I knew that it was not just motherly pride that made me find the overall effect stunning. As I studied each painting, I began to re-see Cindy's life, and I realized that these works of art could help Cindy and me remember together. As poet Anna Walters writes, "It is in remembering that our power lives / and our future comes." The paintings gave Cindy power over the forces that would push her beyond the margins of what our society describes as "normal." "Power over" doesn't mean "elimination of" but when Cindy calls on the languages of color and line to describe her experiences with disability, she becomes an active agent in her own history.

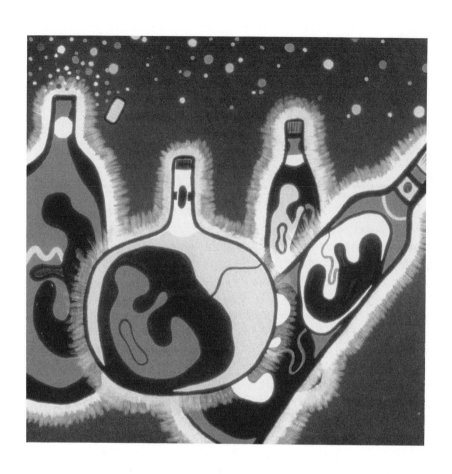

I'm being suffocated by alcohol. Throughout my entire life it's been this way and it will always be this way. FAS/FAE has a mind of its own. I will have FAS/FAE forever till the day I die. I was born alone with this, and I will die alone with this. As a young kid I struggled over and over on one word or one math problem. These mental blocks made me feel insecure and helpless. I feel suffocated for things I can't help. It happens in my own home when I forget the simplest tasks such as refilling the orange juice container or changing the toilet paper roll when I use the last piece. In college I *always* lost my keys, usually three or four times a week. People made comments like, "I could set my watch by you losing your keys." At first it was a joke, but then people got annoyed, and I felt so embarrassed I couldn't breathe. I started leaving my room unlocked. I didn't care if my sound system got stolen, just so I didn't have to humiliate myself once again.

Sometimes it seems like there is an automatic take-over thing in my mind. I will have my keys in my hand and put them on the desk while I pick up my books. Then I'll walk out of the room and lock the door behind me. When I put the keys down and pick up something else, a wall goes up in my mind. It's like the keys don't exist anymore. The same thing happens when I do math. I'll be doing fractions, and I'm getting them just right. But once I get from fractions to multiplication I can't go back to fractions. It's just not there in my head.

It takes me twice as long to do things because I get so distracted. If I'm cleaning my room, I'll look at a dress and start thinking about when I wore it and with whom. Then I'll pick up a magazine and start looking at it. I get lost in the whirl of my mind.

One time a few years ago I was visiting some white friends. I had known this family for a long time and felt very close to them. Several of the young people in the family were about my age, and we had done lots of things together over the years. In many ways they felt like family to me. One evening while I was there, Jeff, one of the young people, came over to visit and brought his girlfriend along. He and the parents got into an argument. The parents were upset that Jeff hadn't returned some equipment he had borrowed from them. Jeff wanted to get out of the house, so he turned to me and said, "Why don't you come with me to pick the stuff up." His girlfriend was already in the car because she had walked out when the argument began. I got into the car with Jeff, and then he said, "Let's stop at the bar before we go to the store." I didn't know what to think or say, so I just went along with it. We stopped at a tavern overlooking a lake and sat on the bar stools. Jeff sat between me and Stacey, his girlfriend, and they both ordered drinks. Stacey ordered a Black Russian, and Jeff ordered a beer. I was so shocked I didn't order anything. Stacey was six months pregnant.

I sat there watching Stacey drink one shot after another. I felt numb all over, and I couldn't talk. I wanted to say "Do you have any idea what you are doing to your baby? That alcohol you are drinking is going to make it hard for your child to learn and to get along in the world. You will pay, both psychologically and financially, for doing this, and your child will pay forever." But instead I sat and said nothing. It seemed as if Jeff and Stacey were not dealing with their baby just like they were not dealing with Jeff's parents. They were trying to run away from everything. I wondered if they knew that I have FAS/FAE.

After I left my friends' house I kept thinking about that night in the bar. For weeks I felt guilty for not speaking out and trying to prevent another baby from getting FAS/FAE. I imagined Jeff and Stacey's child going to school and being taunted for not being able to read. I imagined the child being labeled "stupid" and not having many friends. I imagined the child becoming an alcoholic. Finally I realized that what's done is done. I can't go back and relive the bar scene with Jeff and Stacey. But I will do what I can. In Native tradition we decide things by how they will affect people seven generations from now. I am a warrior, and I need to protect the seventh generation of all peoples against alcohol.

The Native community, as well as the experience of our own lives, has taught Cindy and me about the social nature of disability. Knowing that decisions have implications for people seven generations from now makes us see life in more interconnected terms. When I lobby, as I have done recently, for signs warning about the dangers of drinking alcohol while pregnant, I am thinking of the generations to come. When I explain that FAS/FAE is not limited to one racial or socio-economic group and point out that white middle-class women are at great risk for giving birth to FAS/FAE babies because their doctors are least likely to ask about their drinking habits or look for signs of problems, I am underscoring the ways this disability interweaves the lives of many different people.

Because I am the apparently more able person in this partnership, it would be easy to cast me in the role of helper and Cindy as the helped. After all, I have intervened with teachers, found tutors, filled out forms, written to legislators, established networks of support, and provided financial resources for Cindy. Looking only at this side of the equation, however, misses the ways Cindy has enlarged my perception and influenced my professional life. Art was the class I did least well in when I was in grade school, so I have avoided it ever since. As Cindy points out, with justifiable fury, people in our culture don't have to "prove" themselves in art the way they do in math or reading. I could duck art courses, but Cindy can't escape verbal and quantitative tests. At this writing she is contending with the math portion of the Michigan Teacher Test, and she cannot be certified as an art teacher without it. Only a warrior would face down such challenges.

I have a lousy sense of direction, and I have a very hard time packing or doing any task that requires spatial acuity. More important, I don't "see" images very well. I tend to focus on verbal forms and miss the visual altogether. When we looked at Art Spiegelman's *Maus,* for example, I was so busy reading the language I never saw things like the swastika path in the image of the fugitives or the tattoo on the father's arm when he rides his bicycle. Cindy pointed out these details just as she was always the one to find Waldo in pictures when she was younger. Although I'm still a remedial case, Cindy has taught me a great deal about how to look at the world.

Similarly, I have become a better teacher because of Cindy. I had always known, intellectually at least, that students learned better experientially, but Cindy's study of the Kaska language confirmed that lesson. When she was in middle school Cindy absolutely failed French, and it became clear that she could not succeed at foreign language study in school. The University of Alaska at Fairbanks has a foreign language requirement, and Cindy decided to study Kaska. With the help of a linguist in Whitehorse, we set up an independent study course, and she studied Kaska by interviewing elders, collecting materials for the historical museum, and participating in cultural events. Despite her lack of facility with foreign languages, Cindy learned Kaska because it was embedded in experience instead of decontextualized in classroom exercises. Cindy's success led me to use more "hands on" techniques in my own classes. I now require students to use historical archives, visit museums, and conduct interviews in order to write papers. I have also developed service learning courses which combine a university class with work in the community, and I'm certain that I would not have undertaken this work if I hadn't learned its benefits from Cindy.

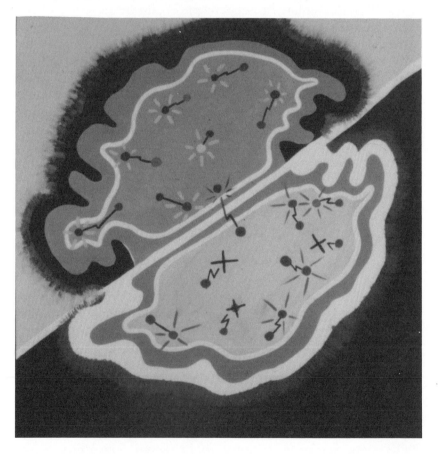

One cold day in the fall of 1995, I was driving back to the University of Alaska at Fairbanks with my good friend Rachel. We had spent the evening with the Walking Hawk Drum Group practicing fancy dancing. As we headed up the hill to campus I told

Rachel about my problem with the dean. I was petitioning to substitute another course for the required math course because I can't do math. "Rachel," I said, "he didn't even read my petition. I don't know what I'm going to do."

Rachel was my best friend at the time. We had known each other for three years, and she knew that I have FAS/FAE. She knew that I had to work with tutors in most of my classes. She knew that I have a hard time spelling. She knew that FAS/FAE makes it hard for me to do many things. But she turned to me and said, "Cindy, I don't understand the problem. Just sign up for a math class and get it over with." I tried to explain again that my disability makes it impossible for me to do math. "Go ahead and sign up," she responded. "It's not that hard. You look fine. I don't think there's anything wrong with you." No matter what I said, I knew that she still would not understand. She would keep on saying that I don't look like anything is wrong with me.

Painting is my way of responding to all those people who treat me the way Rachel did. I got so tired of people saying that there is nothing wrong with me. It feels like they are pouring salt into a wound. I have this disability and when people say they don't believe it, it's like the wound of my disability can never heal. I want to say to them, "What do I have to do, give you a CAT scan?" I thought that people could relate to an image of the normal brain, and I would then force them to see an abnormal brain, something they are not used to seeing. By putting these two kinds of brains together, I wanted to make people think that not everyone has a perfect brain.

One day Cindy and I were talking about the recurring problem of people refusing to believe that she has a disability. "Why," I asked, "do they react this way?" Without missing a beat, Cindy responded, "Because they can't see it." I think she is right. Our culture associates disability with appearance, usually ugly appearance. The hunchbacked Duke of Gloucester in Shakespeare's *Richard III* typifies the way most of us see disability. It is about distortion and deformity. We look greedily and turn our eyes away guiltily, alternately drawn to and repulsed by the irregular or misshapen body. Disability means visible things like wheelchairs, guide dogs, specially equipped telephones, and designated parking places. The invisible disability seems fraudulent.

As Sander L. Gilman, among others, reminds us, aesthetics figures prominently in making distinctions between health and illness. The association between beauty and health finds its dark double in the connection between ugliness and illness.[2] Similarly, aesthetics plays a role in the way our culture approaches disability. We associate disability with the ugliness of illness. Not only is the disabled body ugly, it is morally corrupt. Although it found its strongest expression in the eugenics movement at the turn of the century, the equation between ugliness and disability still permeates our culture.[3] An "invisible" disability like FAS/FAE, then, poses special problems. Because we can't see it, it doesn't fit with our cultural ideas about disability and deformity. Often the response is one of denial.

Not long ago I met Sarah for the first time. The conversation turned to our children and I mentioned having a special needs daughter. "What is her disability?" Sarah asked sympathetically. "She has Fetal Alcohol Syndrome," I explained. When Sarah looked uncertain, I went on, "Her brain was damaged by alcohol before birth so she has a hard time with schooling, making judgments, and following logical sequences." "Oh," said Sarah, and she changed the subject. A few weeks later I ran into Sarah when Cindy was with me. I introduced Cindy, and we chatted for a few minutes before going our separate ways. The next time I saw Sarah she immediately began, "It was so nice to meet Cindy. She is such a pretty young woman. I think she is one of the loveliest looking people I have ever seen. I just can't believe that she has a disability."

Perhaps denial of the invisible disability arises from a deep concern about the fact that disabilities cannot be "cured." Unlike illness, disability imposes a lifetime sentence. As Cindy says, "I will have FAS/FAE forever till the day I die." Furthermore, as Paul K. Longmore observes, disability connotes lack and deficiency, in particular the lack of ability to participate in the democracy of free choice. "People with disabilities provoke anxiety and revulsion because they are defined as literally embodying that which Americans individually and collectively fear most: limitation and dependency, failure and incapacity, loss of control, loss of autonomy at its deepest level, confinement within the human condition, subjection to fate."[4] The medical model offers the solution of "fixing" disabled people, of remaking them. Our experience with FAS/FAE confirms the futility of any medical "fixing," but we remain committed to the possibility of healing.

For us healing is not based on evading fate or fixing but on accepting and integrating.

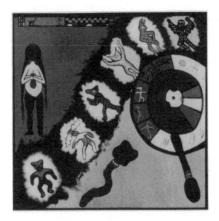 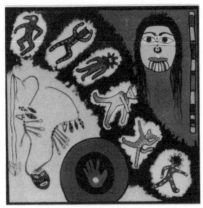

I painted this diptych for all the Shamans of the past who were made to seem evil by Christian missionaries. The images in this painting reflect the same type of power that we associate with symbols of other major religions. I think of the way Joseph Campbell tried to create bridges between different religions of the world. Like Christ of the Christian church, Shamans were healers, and this painting shows a healing path for my disability. Part of this healing lies in telling stories. A couple of years ago I gave a talk in Anchorage, Alaska, in the prevention symposium that the state puts on to battle against the enormous alcohol abuse in that state. After I told my story a Native man approached me. He was recognized in the community as a healer. He said, "If any of my tribal grandchildren have FAS/FAE I won't send them to a doctor, a psychiatrist or even a medicine man. I will send them to you, my young friend." It was at this moment that I learned the message that needs to be sent to the seventh generation. It is that my disability makes me a healer. Like the Heoka in the movie *Little Big Man*, I, too, bring a message of hope and healing.

NOTES

[1]Paul D. Sampson, Ann P. Streissguth, Fred L. Bookstein, Ruth E. Little, Sterling K. Clarren, Philippe Dehaene, James Hanson, and John Graham, "Incidence of Fetal Alcohol Syndrome and Prevalence of Alcohol-Related Neurodevelopmental Disorder," *Teratology*, in press.

[2]Sander L. Gilman, *Picturing Health and Illness: Images of Identity and Difference* (Baltimore: Johns Hopkins University Press, 1995). See especially Chapter Three.

[3]Martin Pernick, "Defining the Defective: Eugenics, Aesthetics, and Mass Culture in Early-Twentieth Century America," in *The Body and Physical Difference,* eds., David T. Mitchell and Sharon L. Snyder (Ann Arbor: University of Michgan Press, 1998), 89–110.

[4]Paul K. Longmore, "Conspicuous Contribution and American Cultural Dilemmas: Telethon Rituals of Cleansing and Renewal," in Mitchell and Snyder, *The Body and Physical Difference,* 154.

GEORGINA KLEEGE

LETTERS TO HELEN

The following is an excerpt from a novel-in-progress titled *HK*.

February 4, 1998

Dear Helen Keller,

Let me introduce myself. I am a writer and sometimes college English teacher. I am forty-one, American, married, middle class. Also, like you I am blind, though not deaf. But I live the sort of life which would have been unimaginable for a blind woman of your generation, a life made possible in large measure by your life and work.

But I am not here to send you dispatches from the future, updates on conditions for disabled people today. I'm writing to ask you about an event in your life which I feel still has reverberations for people with disabilities today. I'm talking about the winter of 1892, when you were eleven, and you were tried for plagiarism. You were a student—the star student—at the Perkins Institution for the Blind in Boston. You had written a story called "The Frost King," as a gift for Mr. Michael Anagnos, the director of Perkins. He liked it so much he printed it in a school publication distributed to benefactors and friends of the Institution. People read it and noticed that your story closely resembled a published story by a Mrs. Margaret T. Canby, called "The Frost Fairies." They questioned you about it, and you denied ever having read Mrs. Canby's story. Your teacher and companion, Anne Sullivan, denied reading it to you. There was not a copy in the library at Perkins, or at your home in Tuscumbia, Alabama.

After a lot of questions, it came out that someone else had read it to you, three years earlier, when you were still learning to communicate with the finger alphabet, still acquiring vocabulary. When people spoke or read to you, you did not understand

147

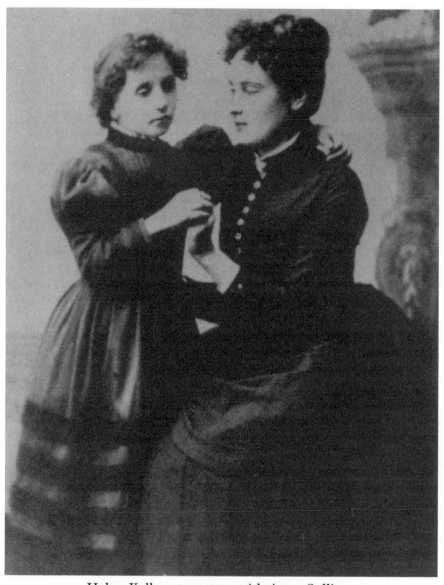

Helen Keller at age ten, with Anne Sullivan
Photo: American Foundation for the Blind

every word, and could not always distinguish speaking from reading, because it was all just words spelled into your hand. So when someone read you Canby's story, you absorbed the gist of it without remembering that it was a story in a book. Then, later, when you sat down to write a story for Mr. Anagnos, the gist of the story came back to you, spontaneously, as if it were your own.

That was the explanation. But the explanation was not quite enough for them. They staged a sort of trial. Anagnos and eight teachers questioned you at length. Sullivan was barred from the proceedings. She was on trial as much as you were. She had achieved a certain level of celebrity for teaching you to communicate, and they felt they had to offer the public some definitive proof that she was not perpetrating an elaborate hoax. They needed to assure the world that Perkins was a legitimate educational institution worthy of private and public support. So they put you on trial. They interrogated you thoroughly while Sullivan waited outside. Finally, they exonerated you. Your explanation became the official story. And life went on as before.

But what made the incident all the more galling was that to prove that you had not consciously copied Canby's story, you had to answer a lot of very tricky questions: "If you didn't copy it, where did your idea come from? How do you know it came from imagination rather than memory? How do you know the difference between imagination, memory, dream, and reality?"

These are questions for psychologists, neurologists, philosophers, not for an eleven-year-old girl, even one as eager to please as you were.

And you were always a little shaky on these issues anyway. Dreams, for instance. Sometimes you woke in the morning and the dream still lingering in your mind would seem more vivid and real to you than waking life. One minute you'd be floating around in a rowboat with your dog Lioness licking your face, or standing on a table eating a bunch of bananas, or sitting in a wild cherry tree feeling a thunderstorm coming up. And the next minute you'd be lying in bed smelling bacon cooking somewhere, and you found it hard to say which sensation was most real.

But the part of this plagiarism incident which bothered you most was the effect it had on your writing. Years later you wrote, "If words come to me too easily it is a good sign they are not my own. I forget them with regret and think of others." When most writers feel words coming too easily they call it inspiration and try to keep at it. "Forget dinner. I'm on a roll."

But what gets me is how during the incident itself, the trial, the inquisition—whatever you want to call it—you just sat there and took it. From all the accounts I've read, yours and others, you stayed calm, cool and collected. You answered all their questions, in full sentences, not so much as a tremor or misspelling. I mean, Helen, get real. If ever there was an occasion to throw a fit, this was it. There you were, eleven years old, accused of plagiarism of all things, with a bunch of adults questioning you with straight faces and at great length about the provenance of your ideas. You were within your rights to overturn furniture, kick a few shins, throw something through a window. If it were me, I would have sat on my hands and refused to answer. But not you. From all I understand (and I guess the point is I don't understand), you just sat there, and took it, answering everything they threw at you until they were satisfied and let you go.

Was it shock, Helen? Is that what kept you passive, docile, and dumb in the face of such provocation? Was it the simple disbelief that comes when what's happening to you bears no resemblance to rational reality? But even so, Helen. You didn't so much as shed a tear. Afterwards, yes, for hours you lay in bed sobbing, wishing you were dead. Eleven years old, wishing you were dead.

Later, you received words of support and encouragement from many quarters. Your old friend Alexander Graham Bell expressed his dismay at the false accusation. Your future friend Mark Twain called the panel of inquisitors a bunch of "decayed turnips" and grumbled that no writer worth his salt would ever claim his ideas to be purely original. Even Mrs. Margaret T. Canby wrote a letter to say she believed you were telling the truth. You felt vindicated by all this, of course. But you must have also felt it was all too easy for them after the fact, all too little too late.

I know you never forgot the incident. I'd wager there was not a day in the seventy-seven years of your life which followed when you did not think about it. It would come back to you out of nowhere, unbidden. There you'd be, sitting at your desk, typing a letter to your editor, or standing on a stage receiving a bouquet of flowers from a little girl, and the next moment you'd feel yourself propelled backwards through time, to your eleven-year-old self, standing in a cold classroom while the air around you vibrated with hostility and doubt, and the being inside you writhed at the injustice and humiliation.

So what I want to know is not how you got over it, because I know you never really did. What I want to know is how you got through it. I can believe shock. Shock I can buy. But you were there, I wasn't. Perhaps you could put a finer point on this, add some detail. I have my reasons for asking. So anything you could do to illuminate this matter would be greatly appreciated.

Sincerely,
GK

February 5

Helen,

Help me out here. I'm having trouble getting my mind around this event. I mean, exactly how do you put an eleven-year-old child on trial for anything, much less plagiarism? But try as I might, I can't let it go either. So walk me through it, Helen.

It's 1892. As near as I can calculate, it's late February, early March. It's Boston, the Perkins Institution for the Blind. I imagine it taking place in a large classroom or maybe an auditorium. Not that they would have invited an audience. But they would want to lend the proceedings an air of formality. I imagine you seated at a large table on a hard, straight-backed chair. There's a larger table facing yours. At it sits Mr. Michael Anagnos, flanked by the eight teachers who are serving as judge and jury. When you write about this later you will note that four of them were blind and four were not. You did not know this at the time. And you never found out for sure which teachers they were, though I imagine you and Anne Sullivan did a good deal of speculating about it. But on the day in question, you don't even know how many of them there are.

Since it is winter and Boston and a large room in a nineteenth-century institution, I imagine the room is cold. Your clothes are stiff with starch. Inside your clothes you are warm and cold at once. A trickle of sweat has already slid from your armpit down your side to your waist. Perhaps knowing that this would happen, Anne Sullivan—Teacher, as you always call her—insisted on the starch. For the same reason, she yanked up your stockings with such force that your toes still feel curled under inside your shoes. She also pinned your hair off your temples with particular tightness, an extra pin on each side.

I know all this because I know what it's like to be a blind child. I know how the idea is inculcated that image matters. All the maternal admonitions about sitting up straight and keeping your clothes clean take on special meaning when the child is blind. "Don't make a spectacle of yourself. Don't be an eyesore." We've all been through that. Your Teacher had been through it herself. She was blind through most of her adolescence, until she got someone to pay for an operation. But her early experience of blindness made her a freak for grooming, yours as much as her own. For instance, she was always on you about your nail-biting, and your habit of fussing with your hair.

Today, she tied a black ribbon in your hair, explaining, "Black shows respect." You always like to know what color things are and what colors connote. Black is for mourning, you thought this morning, but did not say it. Mourning for what, you wonder now. Who died?

So you are there, in a cold room at the Perkins Institution, Boston, February, maybe March, 1892, wearing your Sunday best. Your spine is straight. Your chin is lifted. Your hands are on the table in front of you, carefully folded to conceal your ragged nails. There's another teacher sitting next to you to interpret for you. We'll call her Miss Lawson, for want of a better name. Excuse me if I free-lance, Helen. Your account omits a lot of detail. I imagine her being of a somewhat subordinate status to the other teachers present. Maybe she's a trainee, even a senior student. You know she is there, but she is not speaking to you yet. She does not touch you. The air between you is taut and chilly.

You wish Teacher were here with you, but she is not. She is on the other side of the door to your right, waiting too, probably pacing. She told you this was how it must be. You must go through this on your own. It is the point, she said. To remind yourself of this you keep repeating to yourself, "Leave Teacher out of it."

You cannot articulate it yet, but you sense that part of what's going on today has to do with the fact that Teacher's life here at Perkins is different from the lives of the other teachers. For one thing her salary is paid by your father, and for another she is always with you. The other teachers all have rooms in another part of the building, while Teacher's room is next to yours. Teacher sits next to you in class and spells into your hand and speaks aloud for you. She sits next to you at meals while the other teachers sit at a separate table. She is with you when people come to meet you in Mr. Anagnos's office. Once one of the other little girls said to you, "I wish I had a Teacher of my very own." You wonder if some of the other teachers wish they had their very own Helen.

Resentment is the word for that, Helen. You've sensed it even from Mr. Anagnos. He and Teacher have had a few run-ins—disagreements, they say—about you and how best to teach you. Mr. Anagnos has known Teacher a long time, since she was a student here, back when she was blind. Teacher has told you that they respect and admire each other, but sometimes you've felt something else between them.

So you are here alone and Teacher is outside the door pacing the hall and Miss Lawson (or whatever her name is) sits beside you. She takes your left hand, turns it over and starts spelling into it. "Mr. Anagnos and the rest of the panel have some questions for you, Helen. You must answer the questions as best you can. You must try to tell the truth. You must say what you know to be true, not what others have told you."

I imagine that strikes several nerves at once. Why is she telling you, of all people, to tell the truth. You always tell the truth. Truthfulness is one of your defining principles. And the saying, "I cannot tell a lie," has been on your mind lately. Washington's Birthday and the school pageant were just a week or two ago. But you don't want to think about that now. Now you sense again that they are being unfair to Teacher. Not only is she excluded from the room, but they are talking behind her back. The phrase, "not what others have told you," is about Teacher. At least you think that's what they mean. But you say none of this. You simply spell back, "Yes, Ma'am. I'll do my best."

Like an involuntary twitch, you smile at the front of the room. You lift the corners of your mouth. You show off your teeth. Your head tilts to one side, and a heavy ringlet of your hair slides forward and settles against your cheek. You have a nice smile, a bit forced perhaps, a beauty pageant smile. You can't help it. Your mother told you always to smile when addressing persons directly. But in the same instant you sense this may be the wrong time for smiling. If Teacher were here she would tell you, "Not now, Helen."

Solemn, you tell yourself. It is a solemn occasion. Show respect. Black shows respect. Northerners show respect by looking solemn. You pull the corners of your mouth back to level, and close your lips over your teeth. Slowly, solemnly, not in any way which could be construed as fidgety, you raise your hand and lift the stray curl back behind your shoulder.

Miss Lawson says, "Mr. Anagnos would like you to tell, in your own words, when the idea for the 'Frost King' story first came to you."

You say, "It was this past autumn. I wrote it at my home in Tuscumbia, Alabama. Actually, I wrote it at Fern Quarry, about fourteen miles from Tuscumbia, where my family has a summer home. I wrote it as a gift for Mr. Anagnos's birthday. I wanted to give him—"—"you"? you think. Should you be addressing him directly? Would that be better, more polite? If Teacher were here she would tell you. But she is not, so you stick to the way you started. "I wanted to give him a gift to show my appreciation for all he's done for me, my gratitude for the education I'm receiving here at Perkins."

There is a pause. You know it is a longer pause than it needs to be for Mr. Anagnos to ask another question. They must be talking about something. It occurs to you that these words you have just spoken, "appreciation," "gratitude," are Teacher's words. When you finished the story she wrote these very words in almost the same sentences in a cover letter. Is this what they're discussing now? Do they have the letter there in front of them?

Miss Lawson says, "But the idea, Helen. When did the idea first come to you?"

You have no answer for this. Time is tricky. Memory is tricky. You remember deciding to make a gift to Mr. Anagnos. You remember telling Teacher. She said you should write a story, "a little story" she said, like the ones you'd written for him before, or for your parents, or for class. So you sat down and wrote, "Once upon a time." Words followed. You wrote and wrote. You didn't think what words to put next. They simply came to you somehow. Your fingers moved on the keys of the brailler. The page filled up. Then there was a pile of pages. Then you wrote "the end" and it was done. But you can't remember when the idea came to you, or how. You can't remember thinking about it, making decisions, weighing options, changing your mind.

You say, "I like to write stories which explain things. Like the stories in Greek Mythology." You say this for Mr. Anagnos. He likes Greek Mythology, likes anything to do with ancient Greece and Rome. You have often talked together about these things. You go on, "I like those stories because they help me understand things, and remember them. And . . . " you interrupt yourself suddenly, pulling your hand out of Miss Lawson's as if off the hot stove. You were on the verge of saying, "Teacher was telling me. . . ." You know you must leave her out of it. You say, "I had been thinking about the seasons of the year. Autumn. How the leaves change color and fall off the trees."

But it was Teacher who told you this. About the colors. You knew about the falling leaves already. The leaves fell in Tuscumbia too. You liked to feel them falling. You could stand very still and feel them drifting down around you. You liked to scoop up handfuls of them and bury your face in them. You liked the smell of them, and the smell of them burning. When they raked them into piles, you would run and jump into them. You loved the shifting feel of them as you landed, the way a gust of wind would make them swirl around you like baby chicks swirling around your hands when you threw the feed.

But it was Teacher who told you about the colors. She said that in Alabama the leaves only turned dull yellow and brown, but in New England, where she came from, they turned many colors. She said when it happens the forests would become blazing tapestries of color. Those were the words she used. You had to ask her what a tapestry was. Blazing you knew from fire. The leaves were the colors of flame—red, orange, yellow. Hot colors. But you can't think of this without remembering that it was the first time it occurred to you that Teacher came from somewhere else. You knew that Teacher had come. You could remember a time when there was no Teacher. But you never thought where Teacher might have been before that. When she talked about New England and the blazing tapestries, it occurred to you that she had been somewhere else, somewhere she might wish to return.

But you can't allow yourself to think about this now. Keep Teacher out of it, you tell yourself. Because thinking about her now makes your throat clench and your eyes sting. You say, "I wanted to write a story to explain why the leaves change color in the fall."

Miss Lawson says, "Do you remember reading a story called 'The Frost Fairies'? Or someone reading it to you?"

"I read it last week," you say. Did you read it yourself or did Teacher read it to you? Another bead of sweat forms under your arm and slides rapidly down your side. So much has happened in the last week, so many questions, so much confusion. Did someone braille it for you or was it in braille already? Or did Teacher spell it into your hand? You flutter the fingers of your free hand, trying to remember, to recall the feel of the story, but you cannot. Quick, quick, you're thinking, because they will know this. If you say the wrong thing they will have the book there to prove it.

Last week was the Washington's Birthday Pageant. You played the part of Autumn. The memory makes you wince. You carried a sheaf of grain and a basket of wax fruit, and wore a wreath of autumn leaves in your hair. The night before the pageant, Sunday night, during the dress rehearsal, you were talking to one of the other teachers, and said something about Jack Frost. She said, "Who told you about Jack Frost, Helen?" You said that Teacher must have told you. She said, "What else did she say about frost?"

You hesitated. You actually drew back from her. There was something in the way she said it which made you afraid. Her fingers, spelling into your hand, were hard and unfriendly. It was as if her knuckles and fingertips had turned into tiny iron mallets. Her words bruised your palm and you drew away from her.

Later you told Teacher. She did not speak. She did not move. She sat perfectly still. The flesh of her palm seemed to draw back from your fingers. Then she got up and started pacing.

"But before last week," Miss Lawson asks. "Do you remember reading it before last week, or someone reading it to you?"

"No," you say. "I cannot remember reading it before. When I read it last week it seemed familiar to me. It reminded me of my story. But I do not remember reading it before last week." You pause. There is no human warmth in the air. It quivers. It bristles with energy. But it is not warm. There is no warmth coming from Miss Lawson either. Teacher is always warm. She says she is always cold, but she always feels warm to you. She gives off her warmth but cannot feel it herself.

You know she is out there, on the other side of the door, pac-

ing. You press the soles of your shoes hard against the floor-
boards hoping to feel the vibrations of her pacing footsteps, but
you can't. You know what her footsteps feel like. And when she
paces the vibrations run right up the bones of your legs to your
spine. It's surprising that such a small body can produce vibrations like that. She is small. You're only eleven but you're almost
as tall as she is. When you hug her, you feel all her bones just inside the skin. When you hug yourself you feel more flesh. But
when she paces it feels almost like a big man carrying a heavy
trunk or load of coal. She paces when she is angry. She has been
pacing a lot recently. She is pacing now. You are sure of it. But
you cannot feel it.

And you feel nothing coming from Miss Lawson. You feel
nothing coming from the front of the room where you know
they are sitting. They are not talking then. They expect more
from you. You suck your lower lip between your teeth. Your lip is
chapped. There's a sore spot on the right side because you've
been biting it. You straighten your lips again. You lift your chin.
"I can't remember reading it before last week, but I know that it
happened," you say. Your mouth twitches—almost a smile. "It's
why we're here today."

This may be wrong Helen. This may be me putting words in
your mouth, your hands. It's the sort of thing I'd say. Cut
through the pretense. Make them call you a liar since that's what
they're there to prove. That's me—the hostile witness. You,
Helen, would be more compliant. You may even believe they
want to believe you. And you are always so eager, so hopelessly
eager to please.

You say, "I know that it happened," and let it go at that.

"When did it happen?" Miss Lawson spells.

"Three and a half years ago," you say. "When I was eight. It was
summer. It was in Brewster on Cape Cod. At the home of Mrs.
Hopkins." Is Mrs. Hopkins here, you wonder. You inhale quickly
through your nose, but you can smell nothing, no one. The
room is too cold. Smells don't travel as well in the cold. Mrs.
Hopkins used to be here, you know. She was a teacher here. She
was Teacher's teacher, and her friend. She made Teacher the
dress she wore when she first came to you in Tuscumbia. But
Mrs. Hopkins is retired now, which means she has gone to live in
her house in Brewster.

"It was the summer I first came to Boston," you continue. "The summer I first came to Perkins and first met all of you."

Again your lips twitch. But you stop the smile in time. This is no smiling matter. They may not be pleased to remember when you first came to Perkins. Perhaps what you have done is so bad, they wish you'd stayed away.

"You know that's when it happened," Miss Lawson is spelling into your hand, "but you don't remember it? How can that be, Helen?"

It can be because it is, you think but do not say. Memory is like that. You know you were there. You have been there since. When you go there you remember being there before. You know certain events took place there, but do you remember the events, or only the telling of the events?

What was the question? How do you know but not remember? What a question. It amazes me that you don't call them on it. You know a lot of things you don't remember. You know you were born, but you don't remember that. You know that when you were eighteen months old you got a fever and when it passed you were deaf and blind, but you don't remember that either. Is that in question now too? How are you supposed to know how you know what you know and how you remember what you remember? You're eleven years old. You should say, "Get serious people. Are you listening to yourselves?" But that's not how you operate. You really want to answer this question, really want to prove to them that you acted in good faith, just a little girl wanting to do something nice for the nice man who runs her school, not a ruthlessly calculating plagiarist bent on personal gain and self-promotion.

Think, you tell yourself. "Think," Teacher tells you and taps you on the forehead. "Use your brain." But that is not how you think of thinking. You know you have a brain in there, and that the brain is where ideas, and memories and dreams, take place. But to you, it doesn't feel like the place where you know things. You know things because you touch them. You pick them up. You run your hands over and around them. You know things through your hands, the squared-off patch of palm where words are spelled, the soft pads of your fingertips where you feel the dots of braille. What you know you know as texture and vibration. You feel it in your hands, your chest, the tuning fork of your ribs, the soles of your feet. You taste too, of course. And you smell things. But when you inhale scents through your nose they go down your throat and feel like tastes. They do not rise into your brain.

Miss Lawson touches your arm. You say, "I'm thinking," then add, "I'm trying to find the right words to explain."

Then you say, "Back then I didn't know as many words as I know now. The things I could name were things I could touch. I knew the word for water, but I didn't know the word for cloud." You lift your free hand to point overhead, then drop it, not wanting them to think you don't know there are no clouds indoors. You say, "When people read books to me," you say "people" because it was not just Teacher. It was your mother. It was Mrs. Hopkins. "When people read to me I did not always understand every word. I might understand every tenth word. Even when I read to myself in braille, I did not understand every word. Sometimes I would just skip to the words I knew."

I know how much it costs you to admit this, Helen. You feel shame at your former self's ineptitude. You wish you could claim to have known more then. You wish you had always been the super-star student you are now. I know how much it costs you, because I've been there myself. When I was eleven I lost my sight but I passed as sighted for a long time. I felt ashamed to say, "I can't read that," or "I can't see where you're pointing," because it made me sound stupid.

But this is the price you have to pay, Helen. You have to expose your former self's lack of understanding. That's the whole point. Back then you didn't know, didn't understand.

You go on. "Sometimes, after the person" (not just Teacher), "had finished reading to me, I would ask questions, or I would ask them to tell the story to me again. And I didn't always know for sure if they were reading me the story again or telling it using other words. And other times someone would tell me a story which might have been from a book or might have been made up right there, out of . . .," your free hand moves in the air, fingering it like cloth, whole cloth, thin air, "out of thin air," you say, "out of imagination. I couldn't always tell which was which. Now, sometimes when I read a story on my own it seems familiar to me and I think someone must have read it to me before I fully understood. And sometimes I think it's because a lot of stories are like a lot of other stories. Like stories in Greek Mythology." Again this is for Mr. Anagnos. You want to remind him of all the conversations you've had together, how he always used to praise you, how he called you his special friend. But thinking this makes your lower lip quiver. You suck it between your teeth and clench it. You go on, "I think this is what must have happened with 'The Frost Fairies.' I think someone must have read it to me that summer in Brewster. I think parts of the story stayed in my memory. But I cannot remember it happening."

Again there is a pause. You sit very still. You try not to breathe hard. You feel some movement in the air, small ripples you know are speech. At last Miss Lawson takes your hand and says, "Are you sure this is what happened? Are you sure no one told you to say this?"

"Yes. I'm sure. This is what happened," you say, without a pause, because you must keep Teacher out of it. Though of course she did tell you to say this. She paced back and forth across your room, and then sat beside you and told you all this. The words were slightly different, but there are only so many ways to say some things. But you believed her. You always believe her, because it is through her that you know everything you know. Why would you not believe her? Then, on an impulse, you add, "I did not copy that story on purpose. I would never do that. I know that would be wrong." Because it hurts you that they could think this of you. That he could think this of you—his special friend.

It occurs to you suddenly that you have no way of knowing whether Miss Lawson is really repeating what you're saying. Her hands are so tentative, her spelling so slow. Maybe she's merely paraphrasing, giving the gist. Who is this Lawson woman anyway? You pull your hand away from her and spell into the air. Then you stop. You spell in the air to Teacher sometimes, but you are not sure this is universally understood. You do not know if they are even looking at you. For all you know they have turned their backs.

Miss Lawson's fingers are in your palm again. "But are you sure, Helen? Are you sure Miss Sullivan did not tell you to say this?"

"I am sure." You are determined to keep Teacher out of it. "No one told me to say this."

She says, "Are you absolutely sure that when you wrote 'The Frost King' you thought it was your own invention, your own original idea?"

She says, "Did Miss Sullivan tell you to write that story? Did Miss Sullivan tell you that story and tell you to write it down?"

She says, "Do you remember or are you just saying what Miss Sullivan told you to say?"

"Asked and answered," I want to say. "You're just badgering the witness now." I would be stalling for time, hoping to give you a minute or two to collect yourself. Because, I don't know about you Helen, but this is all getting a bit too fast and furious for me. I can barely keep typing. My hands are cold. I'm actually shivering. You, I can't tell. You are so busy trying to prove you're not lying, and trying to keep Teacher out of it, that it's as if you actually haven't noticed that the questions have taken an ugly turn. The harder you try to shield Teacher from blame, the more central she becomes. And then, what happens to you? Your edges fray. Your core wobbles. You become beside the point, and that scares me. Granted, I have the advantage of a hundred-plus years of hindsight and a more cynical nature than yours, but even so, Helen, even so.

But what scares me more is the possibility that you know only too well what they're doing to you. You feel yourself disintegrating and the only defense you have is to keep hurling back the words, "Don't look at Teacher. Look at me. Look at me. Look at me."

Hold that thought, Helen. Give me a minute and I'll get back to you.

Afternoon

Let's backtrack. Plagiarism. What does plagiarism mean to an eleven-year-old child? It means copying. Copying is bad. When you copy another child's test paper (not that you could do this, Helen) it's bad. But sometimes copying is all right.

When I was seven years old I wrote a story which closely resembled *Black Beauty*. Naturally there were differences. My version was written in the vocabulary of a seven year old, and it included a lot of crayon drawings. But the idea was identical. No one accused me of plagiarism. Quite the contrary. They praised me. Everyone thought it was great—so creative, when in fact, I had created nothing original. And I knew it. I thought it was something I was supposed to do.

Imitation is the sincerest form of flattery and all that. But also,

children learn by copying. Copying is encouraged in certain pedagogical contexts. And not just for children. I'm in the office at
the moment and could pull seven or eight college English text-
books off my shelf which contain sample essays for students to
imitate. If you weren't so busy with other things, I could scan
one into the computer so you could read it for yourself. Of
course, the authors of those books assume college students understand that they are supposed to emulate the form of the sam-
ples, not the content.

In fact, that's how you were educated. You were taught, if not
to copy, at least to compare. Teacher would give you a topic to
write about. Then she'd compare your composition with ones in
books or in the *Youth's Companion* or other magazines. She'd say,
"In the book, everything has a color. You need to say what color
the dog is, Helen. You need to say it's a brown dog." Then she'd
read you a sentence from your composition and a sentence
from the book. You'd balance a sentence in each hand, weighing the words. Then she'd say, "You could call it a chocolate-
brown dog. That would suggest it was a likable dog, a sweet-tem-
pered dog."

At first Teacher had to tell you when and where to make these
additions. Later, you developed a real knack for it. When you
learned that Mr. Anagnos liked everything about ancient Greece
and Rome, you wrote a series of compositions. You wrote about
how the marble columns of the Parthenon were "brilliant white."
You'd learned that brilliant also means very intelligent, very
bright. Inventors like your friend Dr. Bell are brilliant, people
say. You think it's fitting that the Parthenon should be associated
with intelligence. You wrote that Rome was "bathed in honeyed
sunlight." You know that sunlight sometimes feels like a warm
bath, only dry, and that sunlight is usually some shade of yellow
or gold. You like the idea that if sunlight had a taste it would
taste like honey.

Everyone praised these compositions. Mr. Anagnos said your
language was like poetry. But where did they think you got that
language? You have never been to those places. How did you
know all these things? How did you know to put these words to
these things? From books you'd read and things people told you.
How else?

But it wasn't like that with "The Frost King." There was none
of that labored, associative thought-process. You didn't have to

tell yourself, "Add a color here. Put a sound there." It all just happened. You went into a kind of creative trance, and when you came out of it, there was the story all done. You'd like to explain this to them. You thought it was the ultimate goal, to achieve such fluency with the language that a whole story could flow from your head, down your arm onto the page.

But Miss Lawson is saying, "How can you know something happened and not remember it unless Miss Sullivan told you it happened?"

It's not right, Helen. It's just not right. They're not asking you about plagiarism anymore. They're asking you to explain how your mind works, and I don't think that's something a child of eleven should be expected to know. And because you are a child of eleven, you are oblivious to this. You think they're still accusing you of lying, accusing Teacher of lying. So you're arguing at cross-purposes, getting nowhere.

But they're adults and should know better. I try to imagine them sitting there shoulder-to-shoulder, coming up with such questions. I try to imagine him, Mr. Anagnos, your special friend. There he sits at the center of the long tribunal table, the Director of the Perkins Institution, the man in charge. The only man present, in fact. He is fifty-five, widowed, childless. He is a distinguished-looking man, mostly bald, with a full beard cut square around the chin. His correct, somber suit is conservatively tailored. His linen is immaculate. His hands are immaculate. His bearing is at once aristocratic and kindly.

He cannot like what's happening here today. "It isn't right," he thinks to himself. He is an educated and humane man. Why else would he have taken this position at this institution? Some might point out that his coming here when he did allowed him to leave his native Greece at a time of great turmoil. But he is still a humane, compassionate man.

He sighs. He feels the tension around him, the eight teachers who sit at the table on either side of him. He knows which are neutral in their opinion of this matter, which for you and which against. Not that any of them is really against you. You're only a child after all. The antagonism is all directed at Teacher. They all remember her from when she was a pupil here. They know how she is, know her willfulness and her ambition. Some would like to see her taken down a notch. Some bear grudges. And with just cause, Mr. Anagnos would readily admit. She was a handful, a spitfire, as he always thought of her. She was quick, quick-witted, quick-tempered, also headstrong and occasionally disrespectful. Once an exasperated mathematics teacher asked her, "Is your brain ever awake, Miss Sullivan?" and she replied, "Yes, when I leave your classroom."

Mr. Anagnos finds the corners of his mouth curling upward. He lifts his hand to his mouth and coughs to cover this. He was always having to deal with such shows of insubordination. More than once he'd been obliged to threaten her with expulsion and other forms of discipline. But in spite of that, he always liked Teacher. He admired her spirit even when it got in his own way. It made him lenient and protective. When he chose her to go to Tuscumbia and be your Teacher, others objected. Some complained that her own education was too inadequate to qualify her. Others even alleged that she received special consideration only because she was so exceptionally pretty. Jealousy makes people say such things, Mr. Anagnos knows. He chose Teacher because he hoped it would make her settle down, give her a useful purpose in life. And it did. She settled into a zealot's monomania. She has become so prickly when it comes to you, so protective. She cannot tolerate the least question about her methods. She is so young, so excitable. And she has a tendency to exaggerate, stretch the truth. Those first letters she wrote about you from Tuscumbia seemed so implausible. Though she was using methods developed here at Perkins, no one could quite believe the rate of success she claimed to be having with you. "Moderation, Miss Sullivan," he wrote more than once. "Moderate your claims. Moderate your expectations. The child's progress may level off." But when he saw you for himself he could see how easy it was to be caught up in her enthusiasm.

Success had gone to her head, Mr. Anagnos would have to say. She finds it too easy to take full credit for your education. And there's something else. He glances at the door and pictures her out there in the hall, pacing to and fro, hugging herself for warmth, and blowing on her hands. Her face has changed dramatically these last four years, he's observed. Her eyes seem to have shrunk, receded into their deep sockets. This may be a residual effect of her trachoma and the surgeries which cured it. But it makes her look at once haggard and ecstatic, like the martyred saints always look in icons. She is tireless when it comes to you, unrelenting. More than once Mr. Anagnos has had to caution her about working you too hard. "A child needs recreation too," he's reminded her, "an occasional outing, a day of rest."

He sighs. There are those present who have lost all patience with Teacher, and are willing to believe the worst about her. Mr. Anagnos shifts in his chair. He is uncomfortable with this. He is uncomfortably cold. He feels the cold in his joints. The older he gets, the longer these Boston winters seem to him. It is when he most longs for the warmth and sunshine of his homeland. He looks at you, seated there on your hard chair. He likes you. He even admires you, to the extent that a grown man can be said to admire a little girl. You are sitting perfectly still now. Your posture is very correct, he notices. Your clothes too. Your navy blue dress with its crisp collar and cuffs and the ruffle around the yoke is very becoming and entirely suitable.

He likes blind people, having lived and worked among them for so many years, blind children, especially blind girls. They have a certain quality. He likes to see them walking the hallways in little groups, a line of three or four girls, trailing their hands along the wall to guide themselves. They seem so dainty and graceful, like little dancers. There's something ethereal and other-worldly about them. They can be quite pretty, perhaps because they are so guileless and unaffected. He enjoys complimenting them. He'll meet a group of two or three in the hallway and say, "Don't you look lovely today?" And they'll curtsey and giggle behind their hands, pleased to have pleased him, but utterly without pride or vanity.

He looks at you. You are different. You draw attention. There's something elemental about it. It's as if you radiate energy which magnetically attracts the eye. A stranger walking into a room full of children would instantly point at you and say, "Who is that little girl?"

"This is the celebrated Miss Helen Keller," Mr. Anagnos always says. And you hold out your hand and drop a curtsey as you've been taught. You smile, lifting your face to show off your pretty teeth, tilting your head so your hair moves onto your shoulders in a soft mound of curls. You are a delightful child, so cheerful, so pleasing. You demonstrate the finger alphabet. You demonstrate how you can read lips. Mr. Anagnos has let you touch his own lips and throat in many such demonstrations. You always tell him how his whiskers tickle. He feels your strong, eager hands on his face now. He lifts a hand to stroke his beard as if expecting to find your fingers there.

He has watched how people are around you. He has seen grown men's faces transformed by wonder to see you do these things. He has learned to count on you. The most stolid benefactor can melt in your presence, and instantly double, even triple the amount of his donation. There's no denying that you're good for business. Perkins has benefited from your presence here, and not just financially. Now it has the reputation as the finest, most pedagogically advanced institution of its kind in the world, surpassing even the school in Paris. You, Helen, have a lot to do with that reputation. Mr. Anagnos has told your miraculous story countless times, because people cannot get enough of you. In fact, that's the reason he published your "Frost King" story. He'd been a bit pressed, so rather than taking the time to write a list of your recent accomplishments as he usually did, he decided simply to reprint your story so the Board of Trustees and other readers would have a concrete example of your ongoing progress. How he regrets this now.

He looks at you there across the room. People are drawn to you. The light is drawn to you. It's not that you are an exceptionally pretty child. By today's standards you'd be considered a little chunky. But by the standards of your own day, you'd be considered robust and healthy. You're large for your age. Your abundant hair frames your face and shoulders. You have a fine, fair complexion. Your pale eyes are open, because you, like most blind children, have been taught always to keep your eyes open. Your face is lowered slightly. Your eyes seem to be focused on a spot on the floor between your table and his. Not quite focused though. You're not really looking at anything there. It's as if you're remembering something, summoning an almost forgotten image. At the same time you look alert, waiting for something, as if you heard a sound somewhere and are waiting to hear it again. He blinks twice, but when he looks again, the impression is as strong as ever. You look for all the world as if you are thinking.

As if, Helen. As if.

He shakes his head to clear the fancy. Surely you are not thinking in the same sense that he is thinking. He is uncertain. He is of several minds about you. You challenge his imagination, Helen. His reason rebels. No one has ever had to deal with these issues before you. You are only the second deaf-blind person he's ever met. The first was Laura Bridgeman, the first deaf-blind child to learn to communicate with the finger alphabet. But communication for her meant something more modest. She learned to communicate basic needs, basic preferences. "May I please have sugar in my tea?" is the sort of thing she will say. She is an old woman now, still living here at Perkins, in a secluded room on the fifth floor. She spends her days at lace-making and other needle work. Blind females are often very deft with the needle. She reads a verse or two from the Bible each day. At five o'clock she has a dish of porridge or thin soup. That is her life, and she seems content with it—a modest, rather pious woman. Mr. Anagnos enjoys visiting her once or twice a week. She is a soothing presence.

Not like you, Helen. You unsettle the mind. He has stood over you watching you type and more than once had the impression that the words appearing one by one on the page are somehow connected to thoughts as they form inside your head, when he knows it is really a matter of rote memorization and retrieval. You have a prodigious memory, startling recall. Still, it's something like watching the performance of a skillful magician. He cannot believe his eyes. He knows he must not believe his eyes. And yet. . . . Then other times he's had long conversations with you about abstract subjects, classical philosophy, theology. It's hard to call them conversations. He is not particularly adept at the manual alphabet. But when he's found the patience for it, he's marvelled at your ability to ask and answer questions, to refine opinions, to construct arguments. He has actually felt himself communing with a mind as powerful and supple as a grown man's.

He thinks, "Perhaps this will chasten her," meaning Teacher, but maybe also meaning you.

Then he thinks, "This is wrong. It is wrong to subject a child to such questions."

But it doesn't matter what he thinks. Because he published your story this has become a public matter now. Everyone—the Trustees, the benefactors, the general public—will be watching to see how he handles it. Can he really be so gullible, they are asking themselves, to believe that a child like you, stone deaf, stone blind, could actually produce something with such whimsy, such poetry and color? It is easy for them to think the worst of him. He has been here long enough to consider himself an American. He associates with only the best people, the best families, educated and compassionate men like himself, men who value his cultivation, appreciate the fact that he can recite Homer in the original. Still, he is not one of them. He has been Director here for nearly twenty years, but he does not forget that the Trustees originally named another man, whose only qualification, as far as Mr. Anagnos could see, was that he was native-born. And while they praise his work here, he knows that some remember he is only the son of a village baker. His acceptance in their world is only provisional. He knows that the slightest deviation from correctness in dress, manner, or speech will make him drop in their estimation. Or rather it will only confirm what they have always thought, but never said aloud. He has lived in their world long enough to sense the words at the back of their minds.

One snowy night a man coming out of a tavern bumped into him in the street. The man was clearly a laborer of some sort, clearly inebriated. He had to cling to Mr. Anagnos's shoulders to steady himself. Mr. Anagnos could still remember the way the man's hands stood out in contrast to the fine, somber stuff of his own overcoat. They were hands roughened by labor, the knuckles bulbous, the nails ragged and discolored. The skin was chapped and red with a sprinkling of coarse orange hairs. The man's clothes were patched and worn. The skin of his face was ruddy from drink and smeared with orange-brown freckles. His nose appeared to have been broken more than once, a misshapen lump in the middle of his face. The man peered unsteadily into Mr. Anagnos's face. His eyes drifted sluggishly from his hat, to his well-groomed beard to his immaculate collar just visible above his muffler. The man's lips were twisted into a lopsided grin, as if he was about to make a good-natured joke at his own expense, then clap the other man on the shoulder and part as friends. But then the man's vision seemed to clear. He stared into Mr. Anagnos's eyes. The man's eyes were a watery blue, framed by pale lashes. Then the lids squeezed together, and his eyes became sharp slits of icy color. The man said, "Dirty wop," and flung Mr. Anagnos aside with such force he stumbled off the curb into the rushing gutter.

He lifts his hand. He flicks the air as if shooing a fly. He says, "Go ahead, Miss Lawson. Ask the next question."

SARAH RUDEN

STARING AT YELLOW AND GREEN
(LIFE AND ART AND PMS)

Is Pre-Menstrual Syndrome a disability? I never claimed on an application form that it was. Of course you know why not. Who wants to make *that* kind of thing known? Besides, many people would say that PMS is a disability only in the way death is, except that the entire population dies, not just half of the population. Even granted that some women (like myself) have much worse PMS than others, not many disabilities are an exaggerated version of something normal. In the classic "handicaps," there is always something missing or underdeveloped: physical perception, mobility, logic, intelligence—even emotion, in the case of autism. Somebody with more than usual of some positive quality—like emotion—who can't turn it to the social good is merely a criminal. Sometimes PMS *does* cause crime. But I suspect that, as among schizophrenics, the incidence of violence among PMS sufferers is no higher than in the population as a whole. I am a pretty typical sufferer, a couple of experts have told me, and I never assaulted anyone under the influence of hormones. I don't have any statistics to cite here, though. The victims of breast cancer have nothing to complain about, in comparison to us, in the way of the medical research community's neglect.

But I never wanted to agitate or educate. My attitude is what classes me most solidly among the mainstream disabled: I want to work, to be independent, to be judged for my achievement and not for a visitation of nature or fate. If the blind wouldn't envy me for a disadvantage that others snort at if they know of it, they might still envy me for having one I can hide. But then why do I write about it, making mentors and parents and doctors curse their investment in helping me hide it, and making myself calculate what kind of readership this journal has among search committees for tenure-track jobs? Maybe I've been overcome with confessional vulgarity. Maybe that is just another way of describing my curiosity—reckless curiosity, I admit—about how people will react. Print is, at any rate, the least embarrassing way for me to reveal myself, and my most measured way of revealing anything.

Whenever I move to a new place, I look for a doctor who, even if he doesn't claim to know anything about severe PMS, acknowledges that it exists and is willing to give me what I've been taking for it, or something new I've heard about, or something I've tried before. Actually, in the past few years it hasn't been hard to find doctors who will at least fake sympathy; if they aren't convinced that the syndrome is real, they wouldn't risk crossing a woman they believe is using the pretext of a gynecological problem to justify a foul temper. But the latest doctor was so large, so middle-aged, so well supplied with family portraits on his beautiful antique desk, so apparently attached to empirical phenomena, that I thought he would challenge me.

"I don't have many active symptoms now," I blurted, "but I've been hospitalized twice in the past. I always have to take something. It's just a question of deciding between side effects. The injectable contraceptives made me gain all of this weight, so I'd rather have Parlodel, even though it upsets my stomach sometimes. I took Parlodel for a long time in Germany: it's the regular treatment over there. For me, the important thing is to keep excited about my work, and Parlodel doesn't flatten out my mood like the injectables, or like Prozac, but Prozac doesn't even do anything about the clumsiness or the other physical symptoms—"

He was already writing the prescription. "Fine. We know about PMS, though hardly any women who complain have hormone imbalances that show up on tests. But the symptoms can be bad, and they do respond to treatment, so we treat them. Someday they'll find the cause."

I was disappointed. I knew suddenly what I wanted to say to a doctor, and at the same time why I would never say it. I couldn't face a brush-off. I stopped myself from saying, "Look, this isn't about a clinical cause you can isolate. It's about a romantic disposition of the body you people thought you'd discredited a century ago. I have the same hormones acting on me as other women do. It's *me* that's different. Long after the PMS has been treated, I still have thin skin, a sinus condition, low blood-pressure. I'm *delicate*. And my mind works differently; when I was an undergraduate, they used to have fun in the Classics library making me shout by interrupting me while I was reading Latin and Greek. I still can't drive—too little sense of what's around me. I have been monstrously irritable since early childhood. I don't live with my boyfriend now, though I write to him every day overseas; he's a great guy, but I can't put up with the inevitable crap that other women put up with. I used to curse God for not making me a lesbian, but now I realize that even being a lesbian wouldn't solve my problems. Don't any other women feel this way?"

Without saying any of that, I took the prescription to the pharmacy and filled it and went out of the health services building, back to the dorm room where I am staying. It was supposed to be on a "graduate hall," but there are only four or five graduate students out of about fifty residents. One of the two Resident Assistants is a sophomore, and the other one, a junior, wrestled a colleague in cranberries later that term as a prize for collecting the most canned food for a Thanksgiving charity drive. But I love my cinderblock-walled living space with the gouged linoleum. When I first saw it, I had a moment of letdown. My condo in South Africa (where I taught Classics for several years before I chucked it to start over in English) had been big and wood-floored and full of middle-class paraphernalia. I even had a maid there. But the letdown lasted under a minute. I began the most enthusiastic yet of a long series of unpackings, convinced that I had finally made my way to something I really wanted. I was alone. My boyfriend and my parents were entitled to my phone number, I supposed, but if I spent a lot of time in the library people could hardly get at me from day to day, aside from the few hours I spent teaching and in a seminar. I could read, create esoteric rhymes, take long walks and look at colors. I had never been so happy in my life. Was this my disease or was it me? Did I care?

Trance-like sensitivity to color is one of the more specific yet mysterious symptoms of PMS. Others are numbness down the left side of the body (a slight limp of mine becomes noticeable pre-menstrually), and left-hand tremor. The diagnosis, however, is usually based on a "chart," or several weeks of daily records of moods, kept either by a patient herself or by an attending physician. Some women, if untreated, regularly destroy property on day twenty-eight of the menstrual cycle, the day before bleeding starts. Thousands more women have nervous panic that is so pronounced for two weeks a month (or three: certain women's symptoms, like mine, continue clear through their periods), and with such a sharp peak a day before bleeding, that it is hard to believe that the sufferers could go for decades without guessing the cause.

But there are reasons for trying to disregard menstruation and related conditions. I remember a flappy-chinned, fatuous Sunday School teacher telling me—I was ten or eleven—that she couldn't imagine how a woman could ever be president: she herself was simply an invalid during her period; women's bodies were an obvious limit God had placed on their ambitions, as I would soon find out for myself. My resistance to this idea was so strong that it took me years to make even the most basic concessions to what was happening: knowing when I was due, keeping sanitary supplies on hand, remembering to change. The sex-education films and official chat sessions at school, with their emphasis on what was supposed to make girls feel better—wearing grown-up clothes, becoming mothers someday—and with their lack of discussion of what really interested us—orgasms—made other women, in our minds, useless as sources of information about our bodies. We tried to muddle through on our own, hiding our weaknesses with the zeal of Marine recruits, secretly contemptuous of older women for having put up with this for so long, some of us becoming hyper-athletic or anorexic to make it go away. Except in the case of a few gentle, maternal girls, in love with nice farm boys from an early age and marrying right out of high school, we were not on speaking terms with our physiology.

This is how I got to be twenty-five, a Harvard graduate student, in the infirmary with a tremor that looked like convulsions, and blackouts. I had struggled through my second semester of Latin teaching, for several days a month barely able to dial a phone, and losing thirty pounds because of the days I could not focus on the food in front of me. After I was admitted I realized that something like the final stage had happened before: *that* state of mind, the emergency room, the blood on the sheet the next morning.

The way the doctors dealt with my notion of what was wrong, when I could speak normally again (for a few days more, I had trouble finishing sentences) and tell them, reminded me of those conspiracy movies in which the protagonist (always a man—why?) is stuck in a world almost exactly like the one before, only it's the wrong world, an elaborate stage, and no one will admit it. "You're perfectly healthy. You worry too much. Take it easy. Come back for a checkup in a few months," the doctors said.

"I look healthy because it's *this* week. Just wait."

In another week, when my symptoms returned and I showed up as an outpatient, the doctors treated me with anti-depressants; then, when my symptoms got worse, with a higher dose, and then with a still higher dose. Word spread that I was in hysterical denial about a depressive episode, and I could not get another appointment, except with a psychiatrist. My panic and shaking grew. Not eating was bad, I realized by now, but even when I could concentrate on the food I had trouble swallowing because my mouth was dry from the old-fashioned tricyclics.

Finally, a childhood friend, who happened to be a student at Emerson College at the time, took me to have dinner with her in her Quaker residential community. She introduced me to a resident who had hypoglycemia, which produced similar symptoms to mine. She made me listen to synthesizer music. She lent me red pajamas with feet and a pattern of flying bats (she is very short: on me, the legs stretched tight), and we had a tiny slumber party. A few mornings later, she took me to her own fashionable, liberal gynecologist and forced him to see me before his other appointments. I don't think it was anything I said that convinced him, but rather the tampon he found during the pelvic exam: it was from the previous month. I had forgotten it, I explained in chagrin. He referred me to a specialist, who treated me with a restrictive diet: no refined flour or sugar, no alcohol or caffeine. This worked, but was a lot of trouble, and I tried several chemical treatments over the years. I now take Parlodel, which in this country is used mostly to treat lactation disorders. Nobody has any idea why this drug works on PMS.

I have two contrasting images of women from those days. The doctor who treated me in the infirmary was one of those self-conscious professionals, dressed and coiffed and made up as if to act in a hospital soap opera. She said, "What you need to do is eat *three square meals a day*," and smirked down at her notes. The PMS specialist I saw had old clothes and a big behind. There were broken toys scattered around her office and waiting room, for the children of her patients. When I told her the prescribed diet was a hassle, and that I couldn't eat out any more, she sighed and said, "Life is hard for women. I've just been diagnosed with a bleeding ulcer." That news shouldn't have done me any good—other doctors wouldn't have approved of her telling me, I'm sure, and many patients would have been resentful—but it got me started on an important idea: if women have such a bad deal, why do they still feel responsible for everything? Is this feeling part of the bad deal?

I thought about these questions often in Quaker Meeting—I became a regular attender myself, after moving into the same community where my friend had lived (she went to L.A. to work in film)—an appropriate setting. Quakers believe in "God within"; for them, God is located in ordinary human nature and impulses, and it is the worshipper's task to *find* Him, through silence and through the interactions of a community. I was good at the silence from the beginning; I struggle with the community part, much of the time improvising through performances (teaching, singing, cleaning floors so well that people exclaim over them) I can concentrate on in the same way I concentrate in Meeting for Worship. This kind of rattle-trap compromise has been the best I can do. There is no Girl Scout God within me, just a rather morose God designed to do one thing at a time, but doing it well if given a chance. Lately, however, this God is more aggressive, less willing to wait for a chance, more calculating. Last year I spent a week in Utrecht, a medium-sized city in the Netherlands, after a conference, doing nothing but translating the Roman novelist Petronius in the library all day, having the salad bar at Pizza Hut every evening, and lying in a hotel bed and staring at the TV at night. I did not see any sights. I did not want to go home. The Utrecht library had books no South African library possessed, I had explained to the travel grant committee, my boyfriend, the colleagues who were teaching my classes. I consulted those books conscientiously; but it was of more use to my work—and to my peace of mind—that I spent a week alone and single-minded.

Having a disorder normally considered comic, or imaginary, or a form of criminal insanity, has often led me to these half-dodges. When I first found out what the matter was, I told a lot of people, but they didn't want to know, especially those who liked me. They were embarrassed, and they felt that my excitement over finding something organic wrong and my eagerness to treat it out of my life were silly. I had been condemning for years the most interesting forces in myself: I used to envy waitresses and data-entry workers—my hands had always been stiff and unplugged—and bus drivers; at twenty-one, I would have opted instantly for any of these jobs rather than the study of philology I regarded as punishment for my failure to be a respectable, productive member of society. My friends were sick of this attitude not only because of its melodrama, but because it left me stuck in one place even after my diagnosis: by yearning for "treatment," I might as well be yearning to be taller rather than learning to be happy short.

Well, that's true to a degree. With untreated PMS, my emotions were uncontrolled. If I made a small mistake, for example, I might cry, depending on what day it was. I was proud to be able to control my emotions after I got treatment: the sense of being overwhelmed, the fight-or-flight urge, is in fact both organic and treatable. But the emotions are the baseline: they didn't change a great deal in themselves, and the ability to restrain myself, gained so suddenly when I was well into adulthood, brought its own problems. A year after the diagnosis, my dentist told me that I needed a "bite-guard" for my teeth: through grinding, I was wearing away enamel faster than he could believe. A physical therapist recently advised me to rethink the way I walk and stand, in order to save my joints: I lock my knees relentlessly. The sparseness of my social life—and of my room, without rugs or curtains or any appliance but my computer—is not by pure preference, as I may have suggested. Though optimally drugged, I have not been good at handling even the multiplicity and stimulation I want. I don't mean to be funny in reporting that my boyfriend is a doctor and food developer and computer geek with the most expansive, innocent belief in the power of gadgets to create a better world. He has a machine that kneads bread dough and one that vacuum-packs leftovers; he has a newly available clip gun for documents too thick for staples. He went from amusement to horror in finding that not only did I not know how to use a VCR (as in not knowing which way to stick a cassette in), but that I was actually afraid, like an agoraphobic who has had panic attacks in public and decided that being in public is the problem, or like a child who has been humiliated too often through a learning disability and shrinks from trying any longer. We're talking through this—on e-mail, the only part of the Web I'm willing to approach.

But now I come to what most readers would consider fundamental, the question of temper. I did use to snarl at people, and I hardly ever do now, but this change is even less straightforward. I still get angry, but in the case of anger restraint isn't always a matter of piling stress on my body: as an academic, I have other places to pile it, and the system tends to reward me for challenging authority. If I can work out that I am intellectually correct, I come across with such sickening logic and righteousness that it is a wonder I have any friends left—though, when I think about it, my friends are mostly the same people who used to see me crying at apparently haphazard intervals. Maybe they prefer the way I am now, or maybe they just have low expectations. I'm not surprised that I have plenty of readers, since these love sarcasm and polemic. I can see myself ten years from now, batting out the account of how I snatched a religious poem away from a journal after the editor demanded that I change the references to the deity to make them "gender neutral." I didn't react until I was sure I was being principled and consistent and tasteful, and I was generous with the "I-statements" in my letter, letting the editor know why I was upset—but so much *management* of emotion means that I'm never going to forget the trivial incident or put it aside out of shame. I've incorporated it, in that heavy, adult way, and made it hard to grow beyond. There isn't actually a dumber distraction from substantive religious thought than the controversy over gender neutrality in language. But you wouldn't hear me admit this, or anything else, when I'm on my post-PMS high horse.

Another thing readers must be wondering about is where writing comes into all of this. I haven't missed the news that spiritual sensibility, sensory sensitivity, the wanton assignment of meaning to experience, all experience, can be medical symptoms. There is a certain kind of epilepsy that Dostoevsky and Van Gogh were supposed to have had. It makes sufferers hugely impressionable, so that they write or paint all the time, frantic to pass on some of the heavy burden of meaning they take on against their will. Unfortunately, the disease itself does not engender talent or understanding, and a lot of otherwise ho-hum people have had it, and though it certainly increases their interest in themselves and the world, it does not increase their significance, except clinically. Perhaps PMS is like this kind of epilepsy, and this would explain the number of long-haired, middle-aged women in sack-cloth tunics and big beads, making yarn from collie fur on restored spinning wheels at craft fairs. I think I'm more special, I admit it, so much more that I get sick of other women's claims to creativity and long for some kind of standardized test.

On the other hand, I still envy "normal" people, or those without any disability that they've been forced to acknowledge. Their self-forgetfulness must be so natural, so peaceful. They do not have to be conspicuous. As a teenager, I was addicted to looking at color in nature, yet there wasn't a great deal of it to look at in rural northwestern Ohio. I would scout back roads on my bicycle, especially in June when the wheat was young, and chartreuse-colored on low ground. Other discoveries as well fascinated me: a tiny ice-cream truck making its way to a migrant workers' camp on a Sunday, its manic bells the only sound in the enormous flat landscape: a dummy hanging from a tree the day after Halloween; the mere shape and angle of certain farmhouses in their yards. I became known as a writer of bad poetry, and a strange, mesmerized person—and a hiding one, in that I needed to process all of this intake in isolation; in my room or in the hayloft or in the woods, I would rehearse visions again and again in my head, and I hated interruptions. Repeatedly in my mid-teens I lost contact with reality. I would convince myself that a pool of May floodwater in a field was going to stay and deepen into a pond. Or the cloud banks above the woods would start to look like genuine mountains: I would work out some geography in which Ohio had high mountains bordering it, near enough to see. I remember two dreams to which I was extremely attached, replaying them while awake and taking a long time to accept that events in them hadn't actually happened and couldn't happen. In one dream I was floating above the field behind the barn, hanging from several small helium balloons and able to steer myself high or low; for a while I was sure I could take a book up there and read in the sun and wind, as I had before. In the other dream, I walked many days, in great joy and hope, until I reached a city with very steep, very green hills all through it. In certain of my moods, this seemed to be something I could do again once school was out for the summer. The pressing realities of my late teens took away these comforts. The first time I was hospitalized with a breakdown was at twenty.

It might be expected that I do an Anne Sexton riff on women as artists and witches, but in my experience art comes so long after feeling and perception, yet with so little Wordsworthian spontaneity and so much brutal work, that I can't extend my romantic ideas that far. I spend my PMS-free days rewriting my mantic outpourings into what they would probably have looked like if hormones had never intervened between me and readers. Moreover, as a teacher of creative writing and a judge of poetry and essay contests I hold the popular equation of madness and art to be the enemy of civilization and a real pain in the ass. It is better not to be sick. People who are not sick can create beautiful things, and with greater free will, I insist to my students. Maybe I have had some interesting and even eventually productive experiences being sick, but I would rather be well.

KAREN ALKALAY-GUT

ODE TO BOB FLANAGAN

(New Museum, New York, December 1995)

I step into Bob Flanagan's room,
where his parents from Phoenix are sitting by the bed,
and I really should just be satisfied with saying hello
and how much I am impressed by his exhibit—I mean
no body else from the gallery has even dared
to disturb him in his room in the past hour. Yet I
cannot help but persist in my awkward gush
and we shake hands and I look deep into his gentle eyes,
wonder for a moment if his oxygen is really on,
tell him I am a poet too and from Israel and all that
and I am sorry to have interfered with his family chat.

But God, outside this room is the museum of his entire life
of pain—the poem encircling the walls of the gallery, bringing
you into this room through the words as if you must be led by
        the nose
in order to enter a place like this.

By the time I understood
what was going on I was already
inside, the little school charts
explaining the changes of the body,
the x-rays showing the disease
and the nipple ring, the toybin
with the superman doll and the leather
whip, the blocks with just
c/f and s/m letters. C/f for
cystic fibrosis, the stomach aches
alleviated by the pleasure

of masturbation, the pain
of a debilitating disease
cured by pain controlled, directed,
made into art.

Then the coffin with the video of his face.
Suddenly his image opens its eyes as if it knows
we are talking about it. Then the TV screens of his body,
the face at the top, the bound hands and feet on either side,
in the center the genitals the object of continual torture.

He does it much better than I can describe—
so banal my little summary of his world torment
—the text so small a part of it all, just the tip
of a pin-filled, flame-teased ejaculating penis.

ROSEMARIE GARLAND THOMSON

THE BEAUTY AND THE FREAK

The central goal of what might be called the New Disability Studies is to transfigure disability within the cultural imagination. This new critical perspective conceptualizes disability as a representational system rather than a medical problem, a discursive construction rather than a personal misfortune or a bodily flaw, and a subject appropriate for wide-ranging cultural analysis within the humanities instead of an applied field within medicine, rehabilitation, or social work. From this perspective, the body that we think of as disabled becomes a cultural artifact produced by material, discursive, and aesthetic practices that interpret bodily variation. Similar to ethnic or gender studies, disability studies is part of a larger critical methodology sometimes termed "body criticism," which excavates the meanings of embodied differences and explores how the body has been understood over time.[1] Such an approach focuses its analysis, then, on how disability is imagined, specifically on the figures and narratives that comprise the cultural context in which we know ourselves and one another.

The figures and narratives of any representational system are often clearly apparent in the public rituals or ceremonies that produce them. Exaggerated scale, stylized gestures, and intensified signification make such public rituals highly readable.[2] By analyzing the conventions of display and the narratives of embodiment that the beauty pageant and the freak show employ, I will suggest here that the cultural work of these two public spectacles is to ritually mark the bodies on view, rendering them into icons that verify the social status quo. Although one traffics in the ideal and the other in the anomalous, both the beauty pageant and the freak show produce figures—the beauty and the freak—whose contrasting visual presence gives shape and definition to the figure of the normative citizen of a democratic order.

181

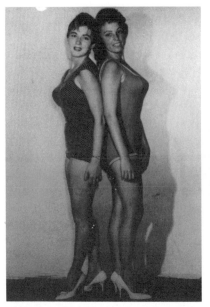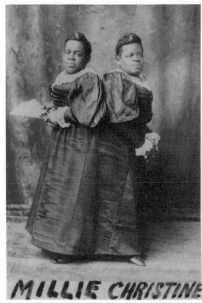

Women on display: bathing beauties and Siamese twins personify the types of beauty and freak.

The highly mediated versions of the feminine body and the disabled body these rituals fashion are elements of an aggregate of rhetorical figures arrayed in opposition to the fiction of the common man, a normative subject position available to the viewers of either the beauty pageant or the freak show.

What I want to suggest, then, is that the dynamics of display and the narrative strategies I discuss here create not only the visually vivid beauties and freaks at the rituals' centers, but that they work at the same time to create an ideal—indeed, an ideological spectator.[3] So, rather than focusing on the actual exhibited bodies or on the responses of actual viewers—who as individuals may indeed resist the assumptions of the exhibitions—I am interested here in examining the beauty pageant and freak show as rhetorical cultural texts that employ narratives, props, staging, costuming, choreography, and technologies to fabricate the cultural figures of the beauty, the freak, and the spectator. In other words, I seek to explicate the dynamics and strategies these theatrical spaces engage to explore how representational systems such as gender, race, and disability operate hyperbolically to create an illusory position of authoritative normativity into which a viewer can enter for a price.

Let me begin by briefly outlining the historical roots of both social rituals. Both the freak show and the beauty pageant were institutionalized in the late nineteenth century as distinctly modern, commercial manifestations of traditional social ceremonies that dated from antiquity. The earliest beauty contests recorded are the fateful judgement of Paris that launched the Trojan War and the Biblical account of a contest that Xerxes held to choose Esther as his queen. Beauty contests descend from pagan Twelfth Night and May Day festivals, which both featured queens, although the criterion for selection was usually not beauty but status. Deriving from Roman spring festivals, these ceremonies persisted in such forms as medieval tournaments, early America's Merrymount settlement, Mardi Gras, the revivals of tournaments in the antebellum South, winter carnivals, and contemporary pageants such as the Pasadena Tournament of Roses Parade—replete with its annual Rose Queen.[4] Freak shows are a modern manifestation of the ancient practice of displaying and interpreting monsters, what we would today call people with congenital disabilities, as ominous and wondrous portents. Reading the bodies of monsters as an index of the divine or natural order can be traced from Homer's Polyphemous through Aristotle, Cicero, Augustine, and Montaigne, through medieval Fools and court dwarfs, early science's cabinets of curiosities, the commercial exhibitions of monsters at London's Bartholomew Fair, Barnum's museums and circuses, and the French scientist Geoffrey Saint Hilaire, who in 1832 coined the term "teratology" to name the science of monsters.[5] Both of these often celebratory, ever astonishing, traditional rituals of bodily exhibition culminate for us today in the familiar, slick spectacle of the televised beauty pageant and the remembered, tawdry sideshow we often furtively visited at the fairs, circuses, or boardwalks of our youth.

The Golden Ages of American freak shows and beauty pageants were more contiguous than overlapping. Freak shows burgeoned from about 1850 to 1920, while beauty pageants flourished from about 1920 to 1970. While both performances exist residually today, neither commands the cultural authority it did in an earlier era. The heyday of the freak show begins in 1841, when P. T. Barnum acquired the American Museum on

New York's Broadway, which institutionalized the previously itinerant exhibitions of monsters—or freaks of nature—that had long gone on at taverns, halls, and fairs.[6] As the nation secularized in the eighteenth century, the interest in extraordinary bodies shifted from religious augury to curiosity, what Constance Rourke calls a "devouring passion for the morbidly strange," that sought fulfillment in the growing entertainment industry and in the ascending discourse of science.[7] Freak shows proliferated in a chaotic, mid-nineteenth-century America that was newly urbanized, geographically as well as socially mobile, increasingly literate, market-driven, and socially stratifying. General rootlessness, a taste for the novel, and changes in work patterns kindled a vibrant entertainment and leisure industry fueled by the ambitions of eager entrepreneurs. The enormously popular nineteenth-century urban dime museums, rural travelling circuses, and the later grand exhibition fairs of the early twentieth century circulated and publicized freaks.[8] Most prevalent at century's end, the freak show began to fade by 1940 as anomalous bodies moved from the discourse of the marvelous into the discourse of medicine, shifting them from prodigy to specimen, from stage to asylum.

Apparently recognizing the affinity between freaks and beauties, P. T. Barnum organized America's first real beauty contest in 1854. Always striving for a middle-class clientele, Barnum tried to mount a genteel beauty contest in the wake of his successful dog and baby contests, but no respectable women submitted entries so he converted it into a photographic beauty contest to avoid displaying actual female bodies to his proper audiences. Although his plan never materialized, a genre of photographic beauty contests emerged that prepared entrepreneurs to marry the beauty pageant with the beach resort industry that developed with the popularity of seaside bathing toward the century's end. Like freak shows, beauty pageants were commercial performances which flourished as leisure, entertainment, and amusement arose from mobility, urbanization, and wage labor. The lifting of restrictions on displays of female bodies, heralded in 1907 by the invention of the swimsuit, authorized the widely popular, cross-class beauty contests of today. By 1925, the female body was exposed, and beauty queens wore suits that resemble our contemporary ones. The Miss America Pageant, established in 1921, institutionalized and fully commercialized beauty contests. As freak shows began to wane, shrinking into the county fair sideshows and tawdry museums, modern, national beauty pageants began to wax and formalize.

The freak show and the beauty pageant thrived within a general culture of exhibition as America modernized and redefined itself.[9] What Mark Selzer terms emergent consumer culture's "excited love of seeing" drove Americans in huge numbers to orchestrated public displays such as Barnum's 1850 tour of singer Jenny Lind, the 1853 art and science exhibits in New York's Crystal Palace, and the 1876 Philadelphia Centennial Exhibition—spectacles that visually sanctified the American political, economic, or ideological status quo.[10]

Spectacles such as beauty pageants and freak shows entail structured seeing. Unlike participatory rites such as Carnival, these visual spectacles enact what Susan Stewart calls "the pornography of distance," by founding a triangle composed of the viewer, the object viewed, and the mediating forces that regulate the encounter.[11] The display's particularly intense capacity to signify facilitates a kind of cultural didacticism where an array of scripts, roles, and positions can be writ large. Although political, ideological, and economic forces ultimately determine the relationship between spectator and spectacle, the mediators appropriate the power of the ritual by choreographing the relationship and manipulating its conventions for their own ends, which were almost always commercial. For example, Barnum—America's master of spectacle—staged the 1863 extravaganza of General Tom Thumb's wedding to Lavinia Warren in New York's Grace Church. This spectacle of what one critic identifies as "the cute" enlisted sentimental ideology, disguised sexual voyeurism, bourgeois attraction to celebrities, public appetite for novelty, and entrepreneurial skills.[12] Barnum profited from this immensely popular and respectable freak show by framing the way the public—which of course extended far beyond those in the church—looked at this notorious ceremony. Similarly, the first Miss America Pageants in the early 1920s exploited the participatory conventions of Carnival and pagan festivals to stage a commercial spectacle that capitalized on the sexual voyeurism of the newly popular seaside bathing culture in an attempt to extend the Atlantic City tourist season beyond Labor Day.

The three constituent elements of the beauty pageant and freak show—viewer, viewed, and mediator—are not equally visible, of course. The viewed object is overwhelmingly conspicuous while the viewer and intermediaries remain obscured. Whether the spectacle is Atlantic City's Miss America in her swim suit and high heels, or the dime museum's Krao, the "Missing Link," or Chauncey Morley, the "Fat Boy," all eyes and all attention rest upon the displayed body so that the complex relationship of looking contracts, seeming to consist of only the exhibited body itself. This visual and spatial choreography between a disembodied spectator and an embodied spectacle enlists cultural norms and exploits embodied differences for commercial ends, creating a rhetorical opposition between supposedly extraordinary figures and putatively ordinary citizens. The beauty pageant and freak show do this by decontextualizing bodies from their lived environments and recontextualizing them within the stylized frame of the particular exhibition, rendering the viewed body a highly embellished representation of itself that reconstitutes its identity. Thus, someone's sister becomes the Queen on her float; black children with vitiligo become "Spotted Boys" in a sideshow; and a woman with a congenital disability becomes "The Armless Wonder" in a dime museum. But the conventions and narratives of presentation make them so. The crown, gown, sash, and float; or the grass hut, spears, and loincloth; or the platform, showman's pitch, and spotlight accomplish this transformation of life into spectacle.

The beauty pageant and freak show differ from many other cultural spectacles because the displayed object is a human body. While sporting events, operas, and political inaugurations, for instance, also involve viewing the body, in those performances the body's actions rather than the body itself carry the significance. Even though beauty pageants and freak shows almost always feature an ancillary performance to enhance the exhibited bodies, the spectacle is the body itself rather than what it does. Cultural resonances lodge in the very bodies of the beauty queen and the freak. So while the Miss America Pageant has included a mandatory talent competition since 1935 and has recently even added a question/answer component allowing the women to demonstrate opinions and intelligence, it is the Swimsuit and the Evening Gown Competitions that nevertheless are the pageant's essence, the vehicles securing its cultural work. In the Swimsuit Competition especially, the generic female body, rather than any particular woman, invites literally and symbolically the scrutiny of an evaluating male gaze, hyperbolically reenacting traditional gender relations as well as confirming masculinity and its privileges. In the freak show, the anomalous body functions similarly to the standard body of the beauty queen by working to establish the borders of the canonical body. Both exhibitions unify a disparate audience into the fantasy of an egalitarian community of citizens and assure them of their status as ordinary and normal.

The dynamic of these performances thus converts private bodies into public exhibitions whose cultural work is to constitute mutually the identities of viewer and viewed by enacting existing power relations. Both the beauty pageant and the freak show traffic in otherness by fetishizing the bodies of people from groups traditionally associated with the body's processes, maintenance, and limitations: women, the disabled, people of color.[13] The presentation exaggerates, stylizes, and saturates every detail of the exhibited body with social meaning. Public stage names, for instance, supplant private family names so that Charles Stratton becomes General Tom Thumb; Fedor Jeftichew becomes Jo-Jo, the Dog-Faced Boy; and Eli Bowen becomes The Legless Acrobat. On the runways and under the lights, Marys, Elizabeths, and Barbaras become Miss Washington, Little Miss Albany, or even The National Potato Chip Queen. Beauties and freaks become tableaux vivants orchestrated to make them hyperlegible texts from which the onlookers can pay to read their own desires, anxieties, and destinies. Although words are certainly part of the textual creation of beauties and freaks, I want to explicate the visual grammar of these exhibitions because that is what generates their primary ideological language. Costuming, props, and staging compose this fundamental visual rhetoric of beauty pageants and freak shows.

The beauty queen's costuming constitutes a sexualized discourse. Consider, for example, her traditional insignia: the satin sash—emblazoned with her public designation and extending across her body—accentuates breasts, waist, and hips as it claims her torso and rehearses the quantification of her body to 36-24-36. Compare this with masculine military insignia, for instance, which rest decorously on the sleeve, the shoulder, the hat. A striking illustration of this literal embodiment of language occurred in the 1964 Miss Antifreeze Contest, which explicitly transformed the women's bodies into an advertisement for the sponsor's product by spelling out the brand name of the antifreeze one letter at a time on each contestant's hip so that as they stood on stage, "Xerex" appeared across the bodies, making them a living billboard.[14] The beauty queen's conventional costume of the familiar swimsuit and high heels signifies potently as well. This contradictory combination of apparel that would never be worn together in everyday life appears on the pageant stage for its symbolic rather than its use value. The suit is not for swimming nor are the shoes for walking. Rather, such costuming affirms the constructed nature of beauty as a form of passive feminine fleshliness. Such costuming is augmented by the beauty's eroticized poses, which instruct viewers on the social position for which she is the icon: a corporeal other for male consumption.

Costuming and props inflect the freak's body, as well. "Armless" and "Legless Wonders," for example, always wear conventional clothing and are featured with quotidian objects such as tea cups, chairs, needlework, or family members. Such staging juxtaposes ordinary trappings with extraordinary bodies to heighten the differences between typical bodies and singular ones. Enhancement of differences is always the major strategy in presenting freaks. For instance, "Human Skeletons" and "Fat Men" often appeared together wearing tights to accentuate their forms. Giants, whose costumes frequently alluded to mythological characters, such as Wagnerian Giantesses, almost always were shown next to people of typical size and ordinary dress. In these juxtapositions, the freak was always individualized by highly marked costumes, such as elaborate military uniforms, while the ordinary person wore a standard, undistinguishing outfit. In another variation of these oppositional images, "Bearded Ladies" in standard feminine garb posed with their husbands to invite the subtle sexual titillation of gender trespasses. Freak shows thus presented people with what we would today call congenital disabilities in order to accentuate their role as what I call corporeal freaks.

The other major category of freaks can be thought of as cultural freaks, who in contrast were usually nondisabled, but were people of color exoticized by costuming and props.[15] "Wild Men," "Zulu Warriors," "Cannibals," and "Missing Links" always appear in generic jungle settings, brandishing spears, loincloths, and the uninhibited hair characteristic of the eroticized "Circassian Slave," a kind of exotic fusion of the beauty queen and the cultural freak.[16] Such props and costumes suggest alienness, transgressive appetites, or forbidden sexuality, and helped legitimate imperialism by depicting cultural others as uncivilized savages needing subjugation or benevolent paternalism.

Costuming establishes a distinction between the highly distinctive beauty and freak and the inconspicuous emcee, judge, managers, and audience. Beauties and freaks appear in ornate, visually provocative costumes that reveal the contours and details of the body, underlining its particularity. The elaborate accouterments and apparel worn by both freaks and beauties embellish difference by marking the body with its own singularity. Similarly, the garish feathers and spears of the exotic freaks highlight bodily specificity, assuring that the exhibited figure cannot assume the universal subject position of the democratic common citizen. Indeed, status and privilege remain unmarked, costumed in the universal gentleman's suit of the judge, the emcee, the showman—the normative male. It is these visually undistinguished figures who signify power now, while the extravagant costumes of the beauties and freaks parody the highly marked bodies of the distinguished aristocrat in a premodern era.[17]

Enhancing the costuming and props, staging explicates the relationships beauty pageants and freak shows try to establish between viewers and viewed. Both freaks and beauties occupy a viewing platform which literalizes their decontextualization, fashions their display, and enforces the objectifying distance essential to the spectacle's cultural work. The beauty pageant's runway typically extends into the audience so viewers and judges can gaze at the bodies from all angles; in addition, the runway's elevation and edges maintain an absolute border between the audience and the displayed figures. The use of floats in modern beauty parades accomplishes similar spatial cultural work by implanting the beauty in a mythical, literally artificial setting that emphasizes her role as icon and removes her from the world of agency and subjectivity. Like the pageant's runway, the freak platform isolates the exceptional, particularized freak from the undifferentiated community of onlookers whose normalcy the freak's presence validates with a body visibly marked by irrefutable difference.

Technologies of reproduction disseminate the choreographed images of both beauty and freak, expanding the arena of their cultural work and commercial potential. Analogous to the platform and runway are the technological choreographies of photography and television, which isolate and project these figures far beyond the spatial and temporal limits of the dime museum stage, circus sideshow stand, boardwalk parade, or gala pageant ball. But where the modern beauty of the later twentieth century is multiple and infinitely iterable as an icon of mass culture, the nineteenth- and early twentieth-century freak who gestures to an earlier tradition of marvelous monsters emblematizes the singular, the anomalously unique.[18] Both on stage and in reproductions, the grammar of freaks appears in the singular, whereas beauties appear in the plural. Such technologies double the effect of representation by literally reframing the freak and beauty already staged by the performance. At the same time, these forms of mechanical reproduction multiply reiterate the messages in the presentations. In the antebellum era, the popular, inexpensive photographic portraits called cartes d'visites and cabinet photographs transferred freak images from the stage to the parlor, nestling them comfortably by the thousands in leather-bound albums alongside familiar family members.[19] Similarly, television shifted the Miss America Pageants in 1954 from local to national communal spectacle, making them universally available by transcending all barriers to seeing the actual shows. In response to technologies' demands, the pageants became even more deliberately structured and began to be staged for television rather than for live audiences. So the camera eroded even the context of live performance from around the exhibited bodies of beauties and freaks, eliminating audience participation, spontaneity, and direct apprehension even as it increasingly circulated the figures of beauties and freaks.

Another aspect of staging is the physical presence of mediators who act as the audience's representatives by directing the action of the performance and providing the verbal narrative which situates the freak or beauty in relation to the viewers. Whether it is the freak show's pitchman, the circus ringmaster, the showman hawking sensationalized pamphlets, the manager arranging the show, the pageant's tuxedoed emcee, or the judge, the mediator is always of the audience rather than of those exhibited. No dialogue transpires between spectator and spectacle; instead, the mediator, who possesses voice, agency, and power, conducts the drama both for the viewers and before the viewers by explicating the intensely visible, mostly silenced spectacle. In beauty contests, judges are, of course, the most authoritative mediators.[20] The relation between judge and beauty institutionalizes the cultural right of all men to evaluate the bodies of all women and recapitulates the competition among women for male favor that unequal power begets. In freak shows, the showmen's role was often augmented by life story pamphlets. These ephemera combined the discourses of both wonder and science by providing elaborate stories that cast freaks as marvels while at the same time enhancing the freaks' credibility by including reports of doctors' examinations or testimonies of scientists about the freaks' remarkable singularity.

Together, these highly theatrical conventions constitute a field of hyper-representation that at once domesticates and exoticizes the freak's and the beauty's exhibited bodies. Even though these practices colonize private bodies by fashioning them into objects of public scrutiny, exhibition does not render them wholly other. Indeed, the freak's and the beauty's cultural function depends upon their being seen as simultaneously self and other, as at once comfortable and strange, as both alluring and repelling.[21] Capitalizing on and amplifying the viewer's potential ambivalence, beauty pageants and freak shows encourage simultaneous identification and differentiation. For example, the "Armless" or "Legless Wonders" who performed mundane tasks like sewing, writing, riding a bicycle, or drinking tea were at once routine and amazing, both assuringly domestic and threateningly alien. "Fat Ladies" and "Human Skeletons" alike dressed like Victorian ladies. Beauty queens at once represent the girl-next-door and the apotheosis of femininity; they are simultaneously highly eroticized and emblems of virginal purity, confusingly familiar and yet teasingly unattainable.

Audiences nevertheless adore beauties and freaks even as they appropriate them, or perhaps because they appropriate them. Spectators pay willingly, watch raptly, display their images in their own living rooms, grant them near celebrity status, encourage their daughters to compete. Moreover, freaks were the most highly paid performers in early dime museums, and Miss Americas of the 1980s could reap $35,000 in scholarships and $125,000 in appearance fees. Distanced yet familiar, freaks and beauties are like pets, existing for the enjoyment, satisfaction, or instruction of audiences who have paid for that privilege.[22] The shows and pageants produce figures that are novel scenery for the arousal or gratification of their onlookers. Through hyperbolized sexual role performances, the figure of the beauty offers to make her viewers into men. By parading exaggerated bodily lack or excess, corporeal freaks invite their viewers to imagine themselves whole. By flaunting savagery, cultural freaks extend the illusion of civilization to their audiences.

We can convey the artifactuality of freaks and beauties by naming these processes of iconography enfreakment and beautification. As an older cultural form, enfreakment uses the grammar of singularity, highlighting the uniqueness of the exhibited body in its difference from the norm.[23] Beautification, by contrast, operates in the plural, suggesting the infinite reproducibility of otherness as a commodity within mass culture. Freak discourse attempts to evoke wonder, what Stephen Greenblatt has called "an exalted attention," which is premodernity's characteristic response to the extraordinary.[24] Pageant discourse, on the other hand, traffics in what Anne Balsamo calls "assembly-line beauty," which is characteristic of late capitalism's effort to standardize, infinitely reproduce, and mass market both subjects and objects.[25]

Enfreakment and beautification illustrate the paradox of social objectification. These processes create a spectacle that renders the lived body's humanity and subjectivity invisible at the same time that it makes the exhibited body into a wholly visible cultural text. The shows and pageants accentuate freaks' and beauties' bodily particularity, while their watchers function as an undifferentiated aggregate. The spectacle positions the viewers in the realm of the universal while it sentences the viewed to the world of the particular. Because spectators only look, do not touch, or interact, or reveal themselves to the spectacles, these are one-way encounters controlled to guarantee the privilege of anonymity for the viewer and to highlight the visibility of the viewed. These are rites of power distribution which license spectators as readers and certify the readability of spectacles. Such a relationship grants viewers a fantasy of disembodiment and forces upon the freak and beauty an illusion of intense embodiment.[26] The figures of the beauty and the freak enter into culture not as agents or subjects but as ultravisible icons, contrived figures whose cultural work is to ritually verify the prevailing sociopolitical arrangements arising from representational systems such as gender, race, and physical ability.

Beauty pageants and freak shows thus ritually enact a kind of symbolic transference of embodiment within a cultural tradition which deeply, anxiously distrusts the body and its vulnerabilities. The dynamics of enfreakment and beautification aim to construct and affirm a normative, generic subject of democracy who possesses the entitlements of agency, volition, voice, mobility, rationality, sameness, and cultural literacy, but who is released from the restrictions and limitations of embodiment. Rendered by the conventions and narratives, the figure of such a normative democratic self haunts the shows and pageants, regardless of whether the actual audience members identify with such an image. Entitled by the dime or ticket and the accompanying leisure his hard work has yielded, as well as informed by the alluring narratives he has read, the figure constructed by the exhibits can freely assume the egalitarian, anonymous position of the "common man." Coming and going at will, this universal subject looks without being seen, judges without being judged, enjoys without being enjoyed, knows without being known. The object of unassimilable bodily difference before him eradicates any felt distinctions from the other democrats who gaze together with him in a communal act of ritualized viewing that unites them as citizens in a social contract validated by the presence of that embodied other. The beauty's ultra-feminine fleshliness, the cultural freak's alien physiognomy, and the corporeal freak's atypical form confer upon them an embodied particularity against which the citizen's body seems to fade into a generality. The intense focus on the body on view offers the citizen the promise of disembodied abstraction, rendering him a kind of Emersonian transparent eyeball. Ritually banishing embodiment in this way soothes suspicions that the body's demands and restrictions threaten unfettered self-determination, freedom, autonomy, and equality—democratic ideals upon which American individualism depends.

NOTES

[1] Rosemarie Garland Thomson, "Body Criticism," *Disability Studies Quarterly* 17, 4 (Fall 1997) 284–6; examples of body criticism include Barbara Maria Stafford, *Body Criticism: Imagining the Unseen in Enlightenment Art and Medicine* (Cambridge, MA: MIT University Press, 1991); Susan Bordo, *Unbearable Weight: Feminism, Western Culture, and the Body* (Berkeley: University of California Press, 1993).

[2] For example, see Mary Ryan, "The American Parade: Representations of the

Nineteenth-Century Social Order," in Lynn Hunt, ed., *The New Cultural History* (Berkeley: University of California Press, 1989), 131–53.

[3]The production of this ideal viewer is similar to the process theorized by reader-response critics through which texts train readers to apprehend the texts they read. Particular readers—or viewers, in the case of beauty pageants and freak shows—might either participate in or resist this shaping. The point, however, is to uncover the practices and strategies that the text employs to produce such a reader. See, for example, Wayne C. Booth, *The Rhetoric of Fiction*, Second Edition (Chicago: University of Chicago Press, 1983); Wolfgang Iser, *The Implied Reader: Patterns of Communication in Prose Fiction from Bunyan to Beckett* (Baltimore: Johns Hopkins University Press, 1974); and Judith Fetterley, *The Resisting Reader: A Feminist Approach to American Fiction* (Bloomington: Indiana University Press, 1978).

[4]For discussions of beauty contests and their history, see Lois W. Banner, *American Beauty* (New York: Alfred A. Knopf, 1983); Frank Deford, *There She Is: The Life and Times of Miss America*, revised edition (New York: Penguin, 1978); William Goldman, *Hype and Glory* (New York: Villiard Books, 1990); Henry Pang, "Miss America: An American Ideal, 1921–1969," *Journal of Popular Culture* 2 (Spring 1969), 687–96; R. A. Riverol, *Live from Atlantic City: The History of the Miss America Pageant Before, After and in Spite of Television* (Bowling Green: Bowling Green University Popular Press, 1992); and Sharon Romm, *The Changing Face of Beauty* (St. Louis: Mosby-Year Book, 1992).

[5]Mark V. Barrow, "A Brief History of Teratology," in *Problems of Birth Defects*, ed. T. V. N. Persaud (Baltimore: University Park Press, 1977), 18–28. For a history of teratology, see J. Warkany, "Congenital Malformations in the Past," in *Problems of Birth Defects*, 5–17.

[6]For discussions of premodern freak shows and monsters, see Richard D. Altick, *The Shows of London* (Cambridge: Belknap Press, 1978); Arnold I. Davidson, "The Horror of Monsters," in *The Boundaries of Humanity: Humans, Animals, Machines*, ed. James J. Sheehan and Morton Sosna (Berkeley: University of California Press, 1991); Leslie Fiedler, *Freaks: Myths and Images of the Secret Self* (New York: Simon and Schuster, 1978); John Block Friedman, *The Monstrous Races in Medieval Art and Thought* (Cambridge: Harvard University Press, 1981); Katharine Park and Lorraine J. Daston, "Unnatural Conceptions: The Study of Monsters in Sixteenth- and Seventeenth-Century France and England, *Past and Present: A Journal of Historical Studies* 92 (August 1981), 20–54; and Dudley Wilson, *Signs and Portents: Monstrous Births from the Middle Ages to the Enlightenment* (London: Routledge, 1993). For discussions of the role curiosity cabinets, early forms of freak shows, played in museum culture, see Edward Miller, *That Noble Cabinet: A History of the British Museum* (Athens: Ohio University Press, 1974); and Arthur MacGregor and Oliver Impey, eds., *The Origins of Museums: The Cabinet of Curiosities in Sixteenth- and Seventeenth-Century Europe* (New York: Oxford University Press, 1984). For discussions of modern freak shows, see Robert Bogdan, *Freak Show: Presenting Human Oddities for Amusement and Profit* (Chicago: University of Chicago Press, 1988); Frederick Drimmer, *Very Special People: The Struggles, Loves, and Triumphs of Human Oddities* (Amjon Press, 1983); Howard Martin, *Victorian Grotesque* (London: Jupiter Books, 1977); and Rosemarie Garland Thomson, ed., *Freakery: Cultural Spectacles of the Extraordinary Body* (New York: New York University Press, 1996). For histories of Barnum see Neil Harris, *Humbug: The Art of P. T. Barnum* (Boston: Little Brown, 1973); A. R. Saxon, *P.T. Barnum: The Legend and the Man* (New York: Columbia University Press, 1989).

[7]Constance Rourke, *Trumpets of Jubilee* (New York: Harcourt, Brace, 1927), 389.

[8]For a thorough discussion of the fairs to which freak shows were attached,

see *World of Fairs: The Century-of-Progress Exhibitions* (Chicago: University of Chicago Press, 1993). For a brief overview of circuses, see Marcello Truzzi, "Circus and Sideshows," in *American Popular Entertainment*, ed. Myron Matlaw (Westport, CN: Greenwood Press, 1979). For discussions of dime museums and the rise of popular entertainment in general, see Andrea Stulman Dennett, *Weird and Wonderful: The Dime Museum in America* (New York: New York University Press, 1997); and David Nasaw, *Going Out: The Rise and Fall of Public Amusements* (New York: Basic Books, 1993). For analyses of the medicalization of freaks in the twentieth century, see Bogdan, *Freak Show*; and Park and Daston, "Unnatural Conceptions."

[9]The notion that performance and spectacle characterize what Jameson calls the postmodern "cultural dominant," which is informed by consumer culture and its attendant commodification, is explored widely in critical thought, especially the new cultural studies. Surely those theories apply to the period and genre I am speculating about here as they coincided with the emergence of western consumer culture that thrived in America, unchecked by previous traditions and nurtured by the ideology of democracy . While I generally am influenced by and draw upon those critical insights and perspectives, I wish here to mount more of a close textual reading, as it were, of the freak show and beauty contest as they function in American ideology than to show how these institutions exemplify incipient postmodernity. See Fredric Jameson, "Postmodernism, or the Cultural Logic of Postmodernism," *New Left Review* 146 (July-August 1984), 53–92; Guy Debord, *The Society of the Spectacle* (Detroit: Black and Red Press, 1977); Hal Foster, *Recodings: Art, Spectacle, Cultural Politics* (Port Townsend, WA: Bay Press, 1985); Janelle G. Reinelt and Joseph R. Roach, *Critical Theory and Performance* (Ann Arbor: University of Michigan Press, 1992); Erving Goffman, *The Presentation of Self in Everyday Life* (New York: Penguin, 1971).

[10]Mark Seltzer, *Bodies and Machines* (New York: Routledge, 1992), 97.

[11]Susan Stewart, *On Longing: Narratives of the Miniature, the Gigantic, the Souvenir, the Collection* (Baltimore: Johns Hopkins University Press, 1984), 110. In *The Society of the Spectacle*, Guy Debord asserts rightly that "the spectacle is not a collection of images, but a social relation among people." However, the limitation of Debord's analysis is his relentless demonization of the spectacle as the totalizing instrument of false consciousness in a hopelessly fallen capitalist modern society. For other analyses of the spectacle in modern society see John J. MacAloon, ed., *Rite, Drama, Festival, Spectacle* (Philadelphia: Institute for the Study of Human Issues, 1984); Rachel Bowlby, *Just Looking: Consumer Culture in Dreiser, Gissing, and Zola* (New York: Methuen, 1985); John Berger, *Ways of Seeing* (London: The British Broadcasting Corporation, 1972); and Kristin Boudreau, "'A Barnum Monstrosity:' Alice James and the Spectacle of Sympathy," *American Literature* 65,1 (March 1993), 53–67.

[12]Lori Merish, "Cuteness and Commodity Aesthetics: Tom Thumb and Shirley Temple," in Rosemarie Garland Thomson, ed., *Freakery: Cultural Spectacles of the Extraordinary Body* (New York: New York University Press, 1996), 185–206.

[13]In a nuanced analysis of the grotesque body, Peter Stallybrass and Allon White in *The Politics and Poetics of Transgression* (Ithaca: Cornell University Press, 1986) observe this paradox of simultaneous marginality and centrality in the representation of the corporeal other; they note that "What is socially peripheral may be symbolically central" (23).

[14]*New York World Sun and Telegram* archive photograph, Library of Congress.

[15]A further explication of corporeal and cultural freaks is found in Bogdan, *Freak Show*; and Rosemarie Garland Thomson, *Extraordinary Bodies: Figuring Phys-*

ical Disability in American Culture and Literature (New York: Columbia University Press, 1997), Chapter Three.

[16]See Linda Frost, "The Circassian Beauty and the Circassian Slave: Gender, Imperialism, and American Popular Entertainment," in Rosemarie Garland Thomson, ed., *Freakery: Cultural Spectacles of the Extraordinary Body* (New York: New York University Press, 1996), 248–263.

[17]For a discussion of premodern costuming of power, see Harold M. Solomon, "Stigma and Western Culture: A Historical Approach," in *The Dilemma of Difference: A Multidisciplinary View of Stigma*, ed., Stephen Ainlay, et al. (New York: Plenum Press, 1986), 59–76; see Thorstein Veblen, *The Theory of the Leisure Class, 1899* (Boston: Houghton Mifflin Co., 1973); and Fred Davis, *Fashion, Culture, and Identity* (Chicago: University of Chicago Press, 1992) for discussions of the signification of dress after the eighteenth century.

[18]For discussions of the iterable image in mass culture, see Walter Benjamin, "Art in the Age of Mechanical Reproduction," in *Illuminations*, trans. Harry Zohn (New York: Schocken Books, 1969) and Siegfried Kraucauer, *The Mass Ornament: Weimar Essays*, trans. and ed., Thomas Y. Levin (Cambridge: Harvard University Press, 1995).

[19]For a complete and insightful discussion of freak photography, see Michael Mitchell, *Monsters of the Gilded Age: The Photographs of Charles Eisenmann* (Toronto: Gage Publishing, 1979). The famous American photographer Matthew Brady, whose portrait of Lincoln was used during his presidential campaign and who photographically documented the Civil War, also made many freak portraits at his New York studio near Barnum's American Museum.

[20]Michael B. Prince, "The Eighteenth-Century Beauty Contest," *Modern Language Quarterly* 55,3 (September 1994), 251–79, argues that the ideal beauty that such contests seem to celebrate is not rewarding to the bearer of the beauty but rather validates the good taste of the judges. My analysis of the beauty contest owes much to Prince's insightful analysis of how aesthetic theory laid the groundwork for the modern beauty contest.

[21]For a discussion of this ambivalence in the process of creating otherness, see Leonard Cassuto, *The Inhuman Race: The Racial Grotesque in American Literature* (New York: Columbia University Press, 1997), especially Chapter One.

[22]Characterizing the relation between pets and owners as one of dominance and affection, rather than dominance and cruelty, Yi-Fu Tuan, *Dominance and Affection: The Making of Pets* (New Haven: Yale University Press, 1984), says "A pet is a diminished being. . . . It serves not so much the essential needs as the vanity and pleasure of its possessor" (139).

[23]I take the term "enfreakment" from David Hevey, *The Creatures Time Forgot: Photography and Disability Imagery* (London: Routledge, 1992), 53.

[24]Stephen Greenblatt, "Resonance and Wonder," in Ivan Karp and Steven D. Lavine, eds., *Exhibiting Cultures: The Poetics and Politics of Museum Display* (Washington D.C.: Smithsonian Press, 1991), 42.

[25]Anne Balsamo, "On the Cutting Edge: Cosmetic Surgery and the Technological Production of the Gendered Body," *Camera Obscura: A Journal of Feminism and Film Theory* 28 (January 1992), 209.

[26]In his discussion of the construction of "typical Americans" in realist and naturalist texts, Mark Selzer in *Bodies and Machines* argues that consumer culture—which was, of course, developing during the period under consideration here—is characterized by "the simultaneous solicitation and disavowal of the natural body" so that some bodies, such as women and blacks, are seen as carrying more embodiment, while others are perceived as being relatively free of the body (50, 61). This is precisely the ideology I am suggesting that the freak show and beauty contest manifest.

DAVID T. MITCHELL
SHARON L. SNYDER

TALKING ABOUT *TALKING BACK:*
AFTERTHOUGHTS ON THE MAKING OF
THE DISABILITY DOCUMENTARY
VITAL SIGNS: CRIP CULTURE TALKS BACK

Editor's note: The following essay discusses the creation of Snyder and Mitchell's *Vital Signs: Crip Culture Talks Back,* a video documentary of disability culture with footage from the University of Michigan's 1995 conference on disability and the performing arts, This/Ability. Released to critical acclaim, *Vital Signs* won the Grand Prize at the 1996 World Congress of Rehabilitation International.

During the ten hour drive back to our home on Michigan's Upper Peninsula, we had plenty of time to discuss how we would compile the raw video footage we'd accumulated into a documentary about disability culture. Three days at an academic conference on disability and the arts at the University of Michigan had left us exhilarated and exhausted.[1] We had left the cameras rolling continuously in the hopes that something revealing would imprint itself on our tape. We remembered the actual filming as a matter of first asking our camera crew of undergraduate film students to carefully frame a parade of academics and artists with disabilities, and second throwing out the most difficult questions in our best pedagogical fashion. We had each challenged our interviewees with all the questions we wanted to answer; they responded in kind with quips and philosophical tidbits from their own lives. We had sought to spar with our subjects in a dialectical fashion, expecting that they would overmatch us and help to create a communal documentary.

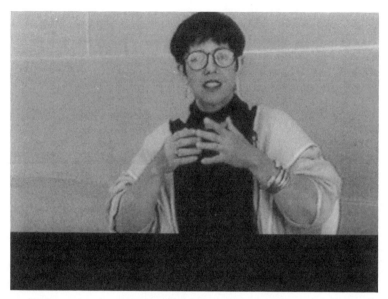

Anne Finger: Let's get one thing straight right away. This isn't going to be one of those movies where they put their words into our mouths. —from "Helen and Frida"

Three weeks earlier, we had originally planned, like good academics, to make a film about the evolution of disability studies and its connection to disability politics. Many of our preliminary interview questions had circulated around university and classroom issues. Yet, as the filming continued we began to suspect that instead we had the rough outline of a film about *disability culture*. We intended our camerawork to reflect that our subjects were in control—masters of their own words, ideas, and images. Of course, years of camera conventions mitigated against these intentions. Hollywood usually situates characters with disabilities in isolated settings at the bottom of a long shot to emphasize their vulnerability or "alien" qualities. Think of the dizzying overhead shots of Annette Bening forlornly wheeling up the city sidewalks of New York in *Love Affair* (1994), or the numerous tracking shots of the sickly and limping Dustin Hoffman in *Midnight Cowboy* (1969) that emphasize his urban-induced grotesqueness. Every would-be superstar gets his or her disability vehicle eventually: Tom Hanks, Holly Hunter, Jon Voight, Gary Sinise, Bette Davis, Joan Crawford, Tom

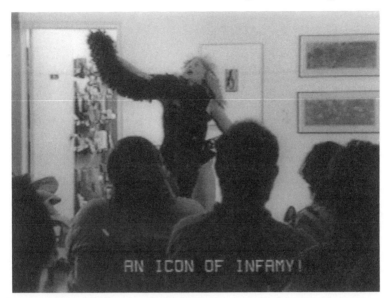

AN ICON OF INFAMY!

Julia Trahan: I am the omnipresent symbol of homelessness, poverty, and despair. An icon of infamy! The personification of hopeless suffering and senseless tragedy.

Cruise, Patty Duke, Jane Wyman, Daniel Day Lewis, Orson Welles, Richard Dreyfus, etc. *ad nauseum.*

Most of all we wanted everyone's image to be splashed across the screen larger-than-life. Near the conclusion of Maxine Hong Kingston's *Tripmaster Monkey: His Fake Book,* her artist/activist/protagonist tells an angry audience of Asian Americans: "A face as big as Odd Job's should star on the Cinerama screen for the audience to fall in love with, for girls to kiss, for the nation to cherish, for me to learn how to hold my face. Take seven pictures of a face, take twelve, twenty of any face, hold it up there, you will fall in love with it" (Kingston 323-4). We sought to make our own subjects larger-than-life. While people with disabilities usually find themselves equated with contagion, undesirability, wasting innocence, or tragedy, our video evokes an intimacy with its interviewees and performers. In this sense, *Vital Signs* embodies a visual revolutionary praxis: get the faces of *our* community on screen, step back, and watch people fall in love with them rather than assume a false repugnance or artificial distance.

Because all of our participants had disabilities—as opposed to

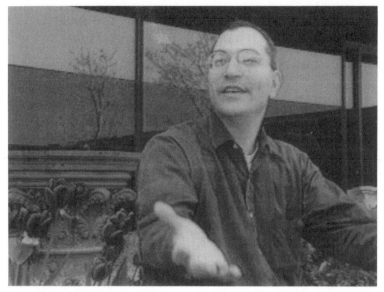

Kenny Fries: It was just given as that's the way we do it in film. And so the whole idea of disability was special effects. It was an illusion. It wasn't a reality.

the staged and performed incapacities of mainstream film and television characters—we saw no need to visually emphasize that fact; instead, we sought to allow our interviewees the choice of "coming out" discursively in their interviews. The visual exposé of physical differences in film and television has traditionally stripped the disabled subject of agency and control of his/her body. We wanted to allow each person the ability to determine the degree and manner in which they discussed their disabilities. Part of this strategy involved providing a space for artists and academics to control the terms of the presentation of their own bodies in their performances, writing, and scholarship. While our taping of the interview segments did not emphasize individual bodily differences, the video centers around the way disability issues affect everyone's life: visibility and invisibility, passing and coming out, accessibility and silence, mainstreaming and isolation, civil rights and public neglect, independence and institutionalization. As a result, *Vital Signs* does not parade disability as a spectacle; rather we sought to escalate the question to a

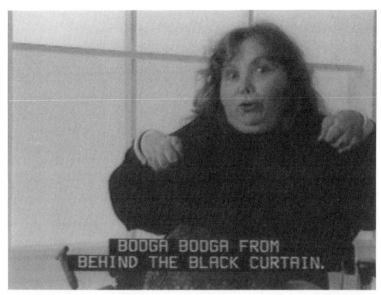

Cheryl Marie Wade: Mine are the hands of your bad dreams—booga, booga—from behind the black curtain.

philosophical level by de-emphasizing the freakshow that physicality so readily becomes in a visual medium.

Since many of our subjects would make their appearances in wheelchairs, we consciously decided to shoot each of our interviews from a low angle. We wanted our subjects to tower over the viewer with their images punctuating their political positions and artistic caveats. When Cheryl Marie Wade, the nationally recognized performance artist of *Sassy Girl: Portrait of a Poster Child Gone Awry*, exclaims, "Mine are the hands of your bad dreams—booga, booga—from behind the black curtain," we wanted our audience to viscerally *feel* the challenge as she displays her "claw hands" on screen. Her flaunting of the cognitive and biological differences which we are taught to hide and dissimulate speaks to the mythic power that bodily variation holds over us. Because cultures have historically sought to erase or eradicate the evidence that the body is dynamic and mutable, the conscious "outing" of disabilities in art runs contrary to this social expectation. The performers in our video refuse the dictates of a culturally imposed isolation; instead they reclaim the terms of the body's

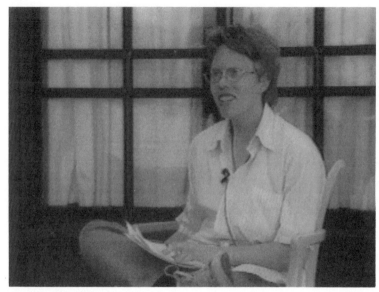

Elizabeth Clare: I practiced the sounds "th" "sh" "sl" for years, /
a pianist playing endless hours of scales./ I had to learn the muscle of my tongue.

portrayal in a visual medium. While talking heads may be routine fare for most documentaries, this is rarely the case for visual
images of disabled people. Both mainstream cinema and news
reportage typically shoot people with disabilities in a way that ob-
jectifies their physical differences—an absent hand stroking the
tire of a wheelchair, the tapping of a cane emphasizing a halting
gait, or the claustrophobic closeup catching the painful facial
grimace of a quadriplegic. Such shots are usually not character
building moments of human complexity; they tend to turn a
prosthesis or an aspect of the body into a metonym for villainy,
excessive fragility, or benighted humanity.

　　We wondered how our on-the-fly, one-take, *cinema verité* approach could provide a space for those of us usually silenced because of unfamiliar speech patterns and rhythms. The "oratory
grace" of well-trained screen icons is achieved through numerous dubbings, re-dubbings, and voice-overs. We thought about
the power of poet Elizabeth Clare's words, "I had to learn the
muscle of my tongue." Our video would try to follow these individual leads. Unexpectedly, our commitment to open caption

the video proved useful for making sure no ideas were swallowed up on the audio track. Such is the irony of the adoption of accessible technologies—everyone benefits. Our video sports numerous technical curbcuts in an effort to enhance access even for the uninitiated.

We used no second takes or rehearsals; all was impromptu and spontaneous. We wanted to capture the emotion and earnest—even belligerent—tone that marks our community's address of issues in need of immediate redress. We felt that common public refrains such as our assumed neediness, excessive dependency, and exorbitant "maintenance" expenses, could only be dismantled with the immediacy of direct confrontation and challenge. The video sought visually to underscore the quotation that stood out in pink neon letters on political-scientist Harlan Hahn's T-shirt: "Piss on Pity."

During the night of the second day of shooting we began to think we had a film. While we had compiled many funny asides and ironic anecdotes about the experiences of people with disabilities, it wasn't until we shot Cheryl Marie Wade's one woman performance that we believed a documentary was taking shape. Watching Cheryl's tour through the disability experience made us both step back in awe of her ability to speak self-confidently about and for disabled people. Only at that point did we start to realize that a film *could* speak on behalf of a collectivity—not because we could capture articulate artists and academics talking candidly about disability (although we did that), nor because film is capable of creating a sense of critical mass (although we think the video does that as well), but because we began to hear a resonance and a repetition in the themes upon which Cheryl's performance touched. Shared points of view and experiences echoed in our minds as a wider cultural commentary about stigma, humiliation, public intolerance, and insensitivity began to take shape.

Historically, disabilities have been narrated as private and individual concerns to be banished to the closets or attics of houses and institutions. We sought to argue that the danger of this social construction of disability has isolated people with disabilities from public view and inhibited them from political organization. The public space of disability has been fraught with obstacles that are simultaneously attitudinal and physical. While the former issue concerns the critique and revision of social ideologies,

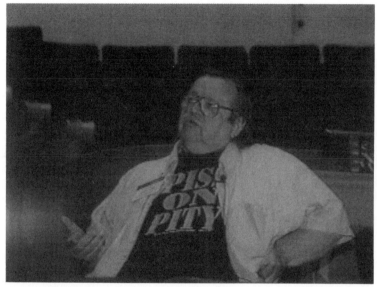

Harlan Hahn: Once we begin to realize that disability is in the environment then in order for us to have equal rights, we don't have to change but the environment has to change.

the latter concern involves an exposé of the ideological coordinates of architecture and the organization of participatory life. This unique combination defines the political program of disability as distinct from other activist movements, and makes the transformation of public space a uniquely literal (and intensely metaphorical) concern for the disabled community.

Because the rental of two cameras enabled us to keep two units shooting over the course of about 48 hours, we hadn't had any chance to get together and allow the project to foment further. During the drive home we started jotting down the memorable images and ideas that had run by the camera on the back of our car's registration papers. Our memories differed as to what was most useable—one of us recalled the Irish artist Mary Duffy's nude performance as the Venus de Milo while the other recalled English-professor-turned-comedian Bob DeFelice's satirical stand-up routine on language. One of us remembered writer and performance artist Julia Trahan's story about experiencing a lifetime of stigma after falling asleep as a child in the back seat of her parent's car, while the other recalled the power of Ann

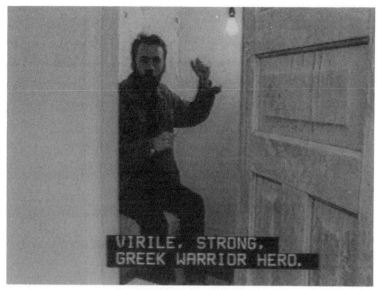

VIRILE, STRONG,
GREEK WARRIOR HERO.

Brad Rothbart: Oedipus is always played as the man of all men—virile, strong, Greek, warrior hero. So he couldn't be disabled. He couldn't have a limp. And to find a director who is willing to re-think not only a concept of theatre, but of the world, is a great obstacle.

Arbor poet Elizabeth Clare's verse on an outdoor balcony on the roof of Rackham Graduate School. We felt that we had been privy to an array of private encore performances and interviews that we could watch over and over again even though the show was technically over. A theatre-goer's dream. All the way home after the filming of the video we had the feeling that we were riding the crest of a political wave that was about to break.

On the one hand, we had thought about how disability lay at the roots of so much artistic production. After all, didn't Dylan Thomas say that "the majority of literature is the outcome of ill men"? (And, we would add, women.) Think of the deformed Socrates and the "hunchbacked" Alexander Pope. Or think of John Keats's consumption, Friedrich Nietzsche's migraines, Margaret Fuller's physical infirmities and "uncomeliness," Henry James's impotence and "back problems," and Stephen Crane's debilitating tuberculosis. Remember the surreal medical imagery in self-portraits by Frida Kahlo, the "sick room" of Harriet Martineau, and the "visionary mad spells" of Virginia Woolf. On the other hand, didn't Kenzeburo Oë argue that one could not truly know a culture until one understood the perspective of its disabled populations?[2] Where was this disabled perspective? Could we access it?

Because "disability" is at best a loose rubric grouping together a panoply of people with enormously divergent physical and psychological differences, our video sought no representative experience or singularizing perspective. The conference at which we shot the documentary proved to be a rather eclectic sampling in that those who attended largely hailed from the ranks of the academy and the arts community. Certain kinds of disabilities such as mobility impairments were "over-represented," while people representing blind and Deaf communities were largely absent from the proceedings. Like the conference organizers themselves, we worked with the individuals who attended the conference; their experiences and ideas would provide a foundation that was an important beginning for our explorations. They could neither serve as "representative" of all disabilities nor could they speak for the infinite variety of perspectives that make our communities vital yet conflicted.

The reasons why some disabilities were over-represented and others under-represented are many. For example, members of the Deaf community do not recognize themselves as "disabled" because they view the classification as still retaining the aura of medical pathology. Instead, the Deaf community has opted for the label of "linguistic minority" which emphasizes their evolution of a separate language and a distinctive set of cultural rituals, values, and forms. On the other hand, a generation of academics with polio and post-polio gained access to higher education partially on the heels of Franklin Delano Roosevelt's presidency, which resulted in a less imposing stigma attached to their lives. In addition, the emphasis upon the value of intellectual and oral agility in the academy does not work against those with mobility impairments to the extent that it discriminates against those who are perceived as "lacking fluency," such as people with head injuries or those who stutter. Just as it is impossible to capture the dynamic variability of any minority group, our video does not claim to forward a version of disability that is absolute or all-encompassing.

Yet, in setting out to articulate "a disabled perspective" we were interested in identifying the coordinates of a politicized defini-

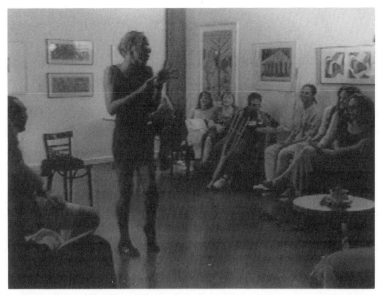

Bob DeFelice: "Broken down" I do not need to be called. "Crippled" was good. Cripples have class. It sounds like Victorian back bedrooms. I like that. It's got mystery.

tion of disability that is widely held. The category of "disability" does not seek to identify or group people who share physiological or cognitive "conditions"; rather it accesses a minority model's definition of disability as socially constructed. While people with disabilities discuss, compare, and contrast the realities of their bodily and cognitive experiences among themselves, "disability" strategically separates the variability of bodily experience from the social meanings which are imposed upon differences from without. In this sense the designation of "disability" signifies an inherently social phenomenon. People with disabilities are first marked or remarked upon by others as embodying a significant deviance from fictional bodily norms. Sociologist Erving Goffman theorizes that an individual with a disability "possesses a trait that can obtrude itself upon attention and turn those of us whom he [*sic*] meets away from him, breaking the claim that his other attributes have on us" (Goffman 5). A "disability perspective" refuses to acknowledge pathology as embedded in the subject and mirrors back the designation of "deviance" as revelatory of that which originates from within the definer.

Although *marked* differences change from one epoch and culture to another, the "disability perspective" we seek to forward in *Vital Signs* developed out of a shared desire to expose the pathological meanings ascribed to bodies designated as outside the norm. Thus, while all people experience fatigue in their lives, the fatigue that people with disabilities experience becomes inordinately freighted with beliefs about their definitive unproductivity, incapacity, or moral lethargy. This fictional correlation between perceived deviance and social undesirability sits at the core of a communally evolving theory of "the disability experience." Rather than identifying a static notion or singularizing narrative of what it means to be disabled, the participants in our video shared an interpretive *methodology*. Our approaches to the world were parallel in the sense that we all understood the necessity of exposing social attitudes as debilitating ideologies rather than as "natural" reactions to tragic realities.

At one point in the early stages of post-production our dean suggested that we donate the sixteen hours of raw footage to our local television station. "Let *them* work with it. You don't know what you're getting into," he earnestly explained. "You don't need the grief." Making and distributing a film would suck up our creative energies and distract from time that could be spent more valuably beefing up c.v.'s (for tenure or for continued employment). While we certainly wouldn't have minded the input of experts, we were suddenly struck with the "inappropriate" nature of our material for public broadcasting. Not just the deliberate nudity of performance art segments, not just the fierce convictions, and not just the footage of poetry and fiction readings—though all these seemed to mitigate against *Vital Signs* ever receiving mainstream attention—we heard this collective, sharp-pitched hum—saw this collective, clear-eyed view—of a disabled people's perspective on society. Who out there would accept that such a shared vantage existed?

Unknown to ourselves, *Vital Signs* would be part of a bona fide movement of film and video in the mid-1990's that would seek to narrate the experience of disability from within the disability community itself. Experimental documentaries such as *When Billy Broke His Head* (1995), *Twitch and Shout* (1995), and *Breathing Lessons* (1996)—all award-winning productions—surfaced alongside our own less extravagantly funded documentary.[3] What these visual productions all shared was a commitment to

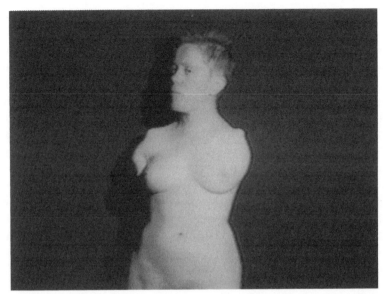

Mary Duffy: The words you use to describe me are: "congenital malformation". Those big words those doctors used—they didn't have any that fitted me properly. I felt, even in the face of such opposition, that my body was the way it was supposed to be. It was right for me, as well as being whole, complete and functional.

telling stories that avoided turning disability into a metaphor for social collapse, individual overcoming, or innocent suffering. They shared a refusal to capitulate to the trite and sentimental productions of mainstream Hollywood films and mass-produced television. Disability—both as a social and individual experience—was coming of age as a full-fledged subject of address and contemplation in an influential visual medium. A common tone and mode of presentation originating from within the disability community significantly contrasted with the traditional ways in which audiences had come to know and understand disability. Instead of seeing people with disabilities as isolated and asocial beings, each of these productions would forward the beginnings of a collective voice.

All together, the voices in our video (as well as the perspectives of the disability films listed above) contributed to the creation of a disability ensemble. Yet, unlike *Breathing Lessons* and *When Billy Broke His Head*, we decided not to resort to a first person voice-over as an organizing strategy for our edited *collage*. Each voice needed to chime in and underscore, refute and counterpoint, the shared tunes of disenfranchisement. We thought of Jennie Livingston's orchestrated montage in *Paris is Burning* (1992)— another narration of the coming out of subcultural attitudes and practices. We thought of Errol Morris's use of an extreme closeup of cinema-house popcorn in *The Thin Blue Line* (1988) to signal distorted and subjective impressions of reality. We even borrowed the idea of title cards with witty dialogue that served to thematize the individual segments in our video from Douglas Keeve's trendy documentary, *Unzipped* (1995), which documented the trials and tribulations of fashion designer Isaac Mizrahi. Experimental filmmakers such as Morris, Livingston, and Keeves generally excised their own personal presence from the "show." Viewers could sense their perspectives on their topics in the structure and arrangement of their images.

Though we did not want to undermine any single perspective, as Morris's and Livingston's methods sometimes did, we sought to show the vital dissent that occurs around key disability institutions and issues. Areas such as language, medicine, and education had structured our questing (and questioning). They would provide multiple fulcrums around which to assemble "healthy" disagreement. As a follow-up to Cheryl Marie Wade's comment that the telethon industry spawns bureaucratic "mega-mega bucks corporation[s]," we inserted Bob DeFelice's irreverent defense of telethons: "As a child I adored the telethon. I would have all my play money out and I'd pile it up on the sofa. And yes, they were using us, we knew that. Even kids understand that they're being used to raise money. But hell, there are worse things than being used to raise money." His childish play resonates in a jest that nevertheless underscores the self-serving rhetoric of Jerry Lewis: "I'm watching children that would not have had a chance had it not been for what we've supplied researchers with."

Once we developed a sense of collective voice, we also needed to orchestrate a collective context. Here we turned to ADAPT (Americans Disabled for Assistance Programs Today) and asked their archivist and videographer, Gordie Hogue, to comb through a history of activist footage such as the historically sig-

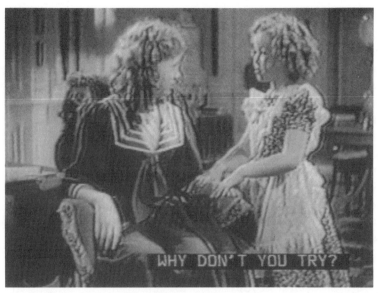

"Your back feels just like mine, and your legs do too. I should think you could walk if you wanted to enough—why don't you try!"

nificant Capitol steps crawl protest of 1989 which introduces the documentary. To highlight our own idea of "distorted impressions" (*à la* Errol Morris) we pulled in riotous film segments from disability lore such as Shirley Temple in *Heidi* telling her wheelchaired friend that she "could walk if [she] wanted to enough—why don't you try!" Other notorious instances were used to document fiction writer Anne Finger's reading from her short story "Helen and Frida": Sidney Poitier handing a pair of sunglasses to a blind girl in *A Patch of Blue* and telling her that her "face looked perfect—no sign of the scars"; or, Jane Wyman dejectedly walking out of the doctor's office with the knowledge that her blindness cannot be cured as the musical score highlights her pitiful fate with a soaring orchestral dirge. Each of these excerpts helps to secure Finger's analysis that Hollywood narratives of disability always "linger on the border between death and cure—the only two acceptable states."

Carol Gill, professor of Psychology at the University of Chicago, most emphatically addresses the idea of disability as a culture: "I believe very firmly in a disability culture, and if we didn't have one we should!" We were driven by our sense of the "newness" of this formulation for many people. People with disabilities occupy a unique relationship to the theorization of culture because our physical and social experience differs so radically from those of other minority communities. Unlike the experience of African or Hispanic cultures in the Americas, the disability community can claim no geographical site or recognized language in a definition of cultural origins. There is no "homeland" or "native tongue" to reclaim in the evolution of a politics based upon an identity of disability. Yet, *Vital Signs* explicitly argues for a growing cultural awareness based upon the experiences of being disabled.

Like other totalizing racial, class, or gender rubrics, disability was initially imposed from the outside as a denigrated social and medicalized grouping. The video identifies institutional narratives to which many people with disabilities find themselves subject at some point in their lives: the telethon's reliance upon the pathos of disabled lives, the medical industry's pathological taxonomies, journalism's penchant for stories of physical overcoming, ethical discourses that underpin euthanasia movements, disease-of-the-week television programs, dehumanizing epithets and myths that proffer the ubiquitous relationship between external differences and internal deficits, etc. The working hypothesis of our documentary derives from our belief that the location of a culture often evolves externally to the group in question, and then must be negotiated by those forced to identify with others who share their political fate.

The redress of this shared political fate led us directly to the dominant theme of the video: talking back. During David's interview with Mary Duffy he found himself using the words—"talking back"—in order to explain our understanding of her poetic diatribe against the objectifications of the medical industry. At one point in her performance she describes overhearing a doctor talking into a dictaphone and describing a dismal prognosis of her future following a medical exam: "as if I had no way of comprehending" my own body's fate. David recalled his own parallel experience in the office of a neurologist when he overheard the examiner say into a microcassette recorder: "patient appears to be in serious repression about the severity of his condition." He remembered wanting to tell the doctor that he had no idea as to the degree of his patients' repressions. Rather than talking back,

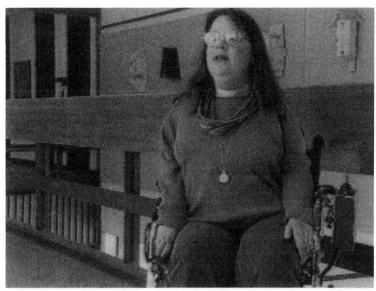

Carol Gill: One of the major contributors to our loss of control is society and the way it views us and its reluctance, no, its unwillingness, to accommodate a different lifestyle—a lifestyle as different as ours—its unwillingness to validate and accept us as part of the human family.

he instead felt silenced by the fact that the doctor could represent him any way he desired—the microphone was his after all. The tape recorder was a reservoir for his own medicalized narratives about his patients—not just a catalogue of diagnoses, but also various pontifications about their psychological states of mind. When David characterized Duffy's performance as "artistic talking back," we thought of it as a kind of child's impropriety to the parent culture.

Just as these doctors (who represented a shared medical attitude even in such different cultures as Ann Arbor and Dublin) could speak at will and without interruption into their tape recorders, we wanted *Vital Signs* to represent a powerful counterpoint. The video became our own way of presenting a disabled people's narrative of themselves without being hushed up or drowned out by other authoritative discourses about them. Carol Gill exemplifies this sentiment when she states: "I saw people in power—the medical and the

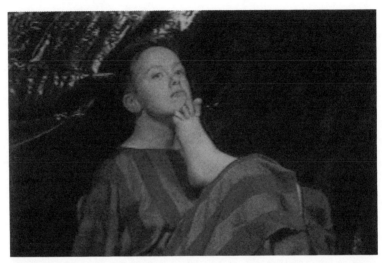

Mary Duffy: I often feel that people react to me as if "you're a walking, talking disabled person—you're not supposed to talk back." You know, people often speak about me as if I'm not there.

allied health professionals—all too often talking about people with disabilities as manipulative, as needing instruction and needing direction and needing to be pushed. That was a big word. They needed to be 'pushed' to do what was right for them. And of course what was right for them was being decided by people who were outside of the immediate disability experience." We tried to construct the video in such a way that a lost agency was recouped—actually it had never been obliterated entirely, but the video sought to capture and preserve it.

Without strong institutions of support for explorations of disability art and culture we struggled to complete the project. Ironically, disability organizations with grant monies refused to fund the documentary because it wasn't "rehabilitative" or "practically applicable" to the real lives of people with disabilities. Film, artistic performances, and writing have not yet been recognized as necessary to a comprehension of a medicalized notion of disability. The central funding organizations for disability research such as the World Institute on Disability (WID) and the National Institute for Disability Research and Rehabilitation

(NIDRR), look upon artistic approaches to disability as existing outside the more rigorous and practical approaches of science and therapy. We sought *revision* while those disability granting operations seek an illusive notion of *correction*. On the other hand, our search for monies to complete the project also led us to discover that funding organizations which privilege filmmaking and the arts failed to recognize the idea of a culture of disability as appropriate to the goals of experimental cinema. Funding operations such as the Public Broadcasting System (PBS), the Independent Television and Video Service (ITVS), and Very Special Arts sought to fund a less multifaceted and ambiguous approach to these questions.[4] Disability struck them as the powerful stuff of first person melodrama, but not as an organizing component of political identity or subcultural perspective.

Funding arrived after the fact from unpredictable sources on the promise that we would only need a little more. For the final edit, we were told that a surgeon at the Mayo Clinic who is also an alumni of our home institution, Northern Michigan University, was deliberating over whether to include us in a bequest to the football program. With no funding guarantee in sight, we sent off final cut instructions to Gallaudet University where a presentable, open captioned version was completed a few hours before it was scheduled to show at a Washington D.C. meeting of the Society for Disability Studies. That night, we found out along with everyone else that our mentally imaged "timing" worked for a wider audience. Elated at every round of laughter, every snicker, every noise that issued forth during the showing, only the next morning did we find out in a telephone call from a university official that the funding for the "edit" would indeed be backed by the Mayo Clinic. We accepted our strange bedfellows.

NOTES

[1]The conference referred to in the opening paragraph of this essay was entitled, "This/Ability: An Interdisciplinary Conference on Disability and the Arts." It was held at the University of Michigan, Ann Arbor, Michigan, in May, 1995. The primary organizers were: Susan Crutchfield, Marcy Epstein, and Joanne Leonard. We are grateful to the organizers, who provided us with the opportunity to film various parts of the conference and interview those who participated. This marked only the second time in history that a conference has been

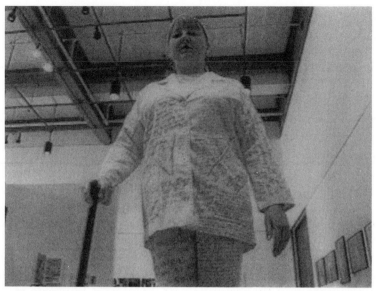

Carrie Sandahl: This piece was really sort of acknowledging the way that I feel that people with disabilities are always situated within a medical discourse. That's why I got the lab jacket and why it's written in red to signify blood And the fascination that people seem to have with a medical discourse of your body—as if it's always written on your body whether you're wearing it or not.

exclusively devoted to work centered on disability from an arts and humanities perspective.

[2]We are grateful to Louise DeSalvo for quoting the Dylan Thomas excerpt as an epigraph to her book, *Breathless: An Asthma Journal*. We are also indebted to her for making us aware of the power of Kenzeburo Oë's philosophy about the importance of comprehending a disabled population's perspective.

[3]For purposes of comparison, a relatively low budget film like *When Billy Broke His Head* received in excess of $200,000, while *Vital Signs* was made on a "budget" of about $9,000.

[4]Since the making of *Vital Signs* we have been told that Very Special Arts has revised its funding guidelines in order to accommodate productions such as disability film and art. Researchers and others are seeking to revise NIDRR's unwillingness to consider work on disability in the humanities.

WORKS CITED

Breathing Lessons. Directed by Jessica Yu. Inscrutable Films & Pacific News Service, 1996.

DeSalvo, Louise. *Breathless: An Asthma Journal*. Boston: Beacon Press, 1997.

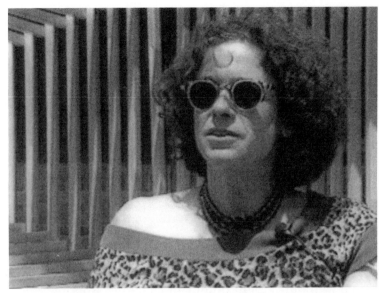

Simi Linton: And I went off and went back to my apartment and spent the next four months in Berkeley just exploring the pleasure and the fun of life as a disabled woman."

Goffman, Erving. *Stigma: Notes on the Management of Spoiled Identity.* Englewood Cliffs, NJ: Prentice Hall, 1963.

Kingston, Maxine Hong. *Tripmaster Monkey: His Fake Book.* New York: Alfred A. Knopf, 1989.

Twitch and Shout. Directed by Lauren Chiten. PBS, 1995.

Vital Signs: Crip Culture Talks Back. Directed by Sharon L. Snyder and David T. Mitchell. Brace Yourselves Productions. Northern Michigan, 1996.

When Billy Broke His Head. Directed by Billy Golfus. ITVS, 1995.

SUSAN E. FERNBACH

WHEELCHAIR
OR
MARKO TAKES LIFE LYING DOWN

1

It was a carrot, and a stick. If he could drive it,
He could go to college. So even though the dreaded 50s virus
Left him with only a right thumb and a left leg working,
No exception was made. Sitting up, he started to suffocate,
So he lay down, learned to drive, looked into a mirror to see
Where he was headed, pushed a lever with his foot to stop,
Let up to go, steered with his ankle, sometimes circled endlessly
Before a sidewalk ramp. Once he caught himself on the roots
Of a Telegraph Avenue street tree, and got a boost from an
Unknown Benz driver. He lusted after the women who cared
For his body, braved the stares and the daily struggle,
Contemplated quitting so he wouldn't have to drive the chair.
But he learned to write and to love words, and graduated
To cheers and applause and flashbulbs and TV cameras.
One day he dumped himself over onto an unforgiving sidewalk.
After the curious crowds and the paramedics and the
     ambulance
And the long defeated sobs, the fear never left him.
He never drove the chair again.

2

It was a still vehicle in the best sense, allowing him
To taste the world, even though he was
Perpendicular to everyone and nearly
Every thing. He went to parties where he gazed

218

At crotches and asses all evening, screamed himself
Hoarse in windy Candlestick Park, lusted after
The women who cared for his body and pushed
His chair. He savored tea in the Japanese garden,
Took graduate courses, lusted after the men
Who cared for his body and pushed his chair. He
Wrote stories and poems, joined a writing group,
Raged, obsessed, and one day, cooked his brains
And body at an outdoor Shakespeare play. After
The vomiting and the dehydration and the IVs
And the coma, the weakness never left him. He
Never spent more than two hours in a chair again.

3

Now it is used so infrequently—
Brief terror-laced outings
To the bookstore, the dentist,
Optometrist, the park—
That dust collects.
Now its portable oxygen stands
Ready to keep him alive
Should electricity fail.
Now he pecks out his life story,
Gives reporters their interviews. He
Receives letters from all over the world,
Reads accolades that salute him
For being alive still—
It's been four decades since the vaccine.
Now he's too tired to be very angry.
Now the dross has been burned away.
He has a lover now, after all this time.
Their hearts, and minds,
Sometimes their hands, entwine
Like one of those old wooden puzzles
He watched his little brother play with.
Like their bodies never will.
She calls the chair Old Faithful,
And on the rare occasions that
She spends the night,
He sees it draped with her clothes.

FLOYD SKLOOT

SELF-PORTRAIT WITH
1911 NY YANKEES CAP

The subtlest approach would be to ignore
the gray wool cap with its halo of air
vents, its navy blue button, monogram
and bill. The rounded, crownless fit and air
of slapdash speed should also be ignored
so that the grandeur of the monogram

can assert itself. Of course the Yankees
in 1911 were a weak team
best known for hitting triples and stealing
bases. They were a shadow of the teams
that later came to rule baseball, Yankee
teams who began their greatness by stealing

Babe Ruth from the Red Sox January
third, 1920. Little Birdie Cree
was the kind of player who wore this cap.
Although a true wizard with the bat, Cree
kept getting hurt and in January
of 1916 relinquished his cap

and flannels for good to settle beside
the Susquehanna and work in machine
parts. Birdie was my size, too small to play
every day. The body is a machine
after all, and must fit its tasks. Besides,
Cree was temperamental, someone who played

hard, I imagine from his statistics,
and did not consider that his body
might give out. Medical science was far
behind where it is now, when the body
seems to yield its secrets and statistics
to tell us with grave certainty how far

we have let ourselves drift from perfect health.
Yet medical science cannot today
explain how a virus that found its way
to my brain six years ago can today
be responsible for my shattered health
or how my thoughts get lost along the way

whenever I deal with abstract ideas.
In the mirror, the old cap I forgot
I was wearing gives me a new idea
which, as I turn to note it, I forget.

JOAN SELIGER SIDNEY

LAPS

In this marriage of water and air
always she is the beginner

teaching her hands and arms
to push away the water, to raise

her head, to breathe. Though
she swims her laps, butterflying

up and back, trying to kick loose
her leg muscles, the hamstrings

spasm, then left foot crosses right,
forces her to invent a one-legged

way to swim. No more can she
hoist her body out of the pool, or

climb the metal stairs. Instead
she sits in the hydraulic chair, waits

for someone to flick the switch,
and lets technology take her.

Immobile in air
gravity reclaims her body.

In the locker room, there's
always a woman to pull up

her panties, stretch slacks, socks.
After years of early-bird swims

they know each other's bodies.
Wrinkling skin, diminishing limbs.

Nothing holds them back. Lap
by lap their hands part the water.

ROBYN SARAH

WAITING FOR THE OPERATION

The letters began arriving around 1986. Addressed at first to my
husband, with whom I'd co-founded a small literary press, the
earliest ones were handwritten in ballpoint pen; later, some
came addressed to me, and they were typed, photocopied. Sometimes they were photocopies of photocopies, the print grown
faint. Enclosed with them were fuzzy copies of press clippings,
articles from medical journals. Every five or six months a new
one would arrive, with slight variations updating the text, but the
message essentially the same: a personal appeal for help, a plea
to send money. *For the past several years, I have been suffering with
a severe case of Parkinson's Disease. My condition has deteriorated to the
point where I am almost completely paralyzed and require 24-hour care.
. . . You see, if I am not moved every few minutes from a lying to a sitting position and back again, my throat and chest muscles tighten
around me like a vise, making it almost impossible to breathe. . . . My
only hope for survival is a new form of cell transplant surgery not yet
available in Canada. . . . The operation is expensive; with travel expenses, the cost will come to $35,000. . . .*
The author of the letters, Ken Hertz, was not unknown to us,
though our contacts had been infrequent and only peripheral in
the Montreal literary community. We knew he'd been a poet
prodigy in the 1960s, when his poems—written between the ages
of 13 and 19—had been widely published in Canadian literary
journals, attracting the attention of established poets who
likened him to Rimbaud. We knew that in the 1970s he and fel-
low-poet Seymour Mayne had founded a small press, Ingluvin
Publications—an outgrowth of their magazine Ingluvin, which
had featured work by the young Leonard Cohen, among others.
Then it seemed his writing and publishing dropped off, though
he continued to move in literary circles. We'd heard through the
grapevine that he'd been stricken with Parkinson's in the early

1980s, while still in his thirties. But at the time his first letters arrived, informing us of the severity of his condition, our marriage was on the rocks—and financial strain was one of the things that had put it there. We were not in a position to help.

In the spring of 1987, with the support of some prominent names in the arts, Hertz managed to raise the money to fly to Mexico City for pioneering adrenal-cell surgery. After extensive testing, he was found too weak to operate on, and was flown home. But not long after, the letters resumed. Now, Hertz informed us, a less invasive technique had been developed, involving a transplant of cells from aborted fetuses (rather than the patient's own adrenal cells). *I have contacted . . . the first neurologist to perform the fetal-cell implant operation in the United States. After conferring with my neurologist in Montreal, he has agreed to accept me as a candidate. . . . The operation, which is not yet covered under the Quebec health plan, will be expensive, $30,000 U.S. . . . I have already raised two-thirds of the funds, but without further assistance I will not be able to have the operation I so desperately need. . . . Can you help?*

From the start, there was something disquieting, something almost shady, about the letters. Was it that they came from an individual (and more or less a stranger) rather than an organization; from an obscure home address—7041 Ostell Crescent—rather than some suite in a downtown office building? Was it the smudged photocopies—the text that had been typed, sometimes with strikeovers, on a manual typewriter, and signed (by whom, actually?) "(for) Ken Hertz," in green ballpoint? Was it the idea that this man was campaigning on his own behalf for private donations to pay for an experimental procedure which—if one bothered to read the accompanying literature—was not only extremely expensive, but did not guarantee results? And if the author was, as he described himself, truly paralyzed and virtually unable to speak—then who had written and typed the letters? Who had made the photocopies, addressed the envelopes, compiled and stamped and mailed the fund-raising packages? Who was providing the in-home care that involved moving this bedridden body every few minutes, around the clock, for months upon months . . . years upon years? Family, friends, volunteers . . . organized in shifts? How long could they keep that up? It was barely imaginable. It was too disturbing to contemplate.

My marriage collapsed in the spring of 1988. Alone with two children and no support payments—teaching at two schools while at the same time trying to keep up with the needs of ailing grandparents—I continued to receive Hertz's personal appeals. Adversity made it hard not to respond. Once in a while, instead of cashing the Quebec government's token $25 monthly "family allowance" check, I'd sign it over to Ken Hertz and drop it in the mail. An extra $25 wasn't going to make my life significantly easier this month, I'd reason, but every penny probably counted for Hertz. And then conscience would cross-question me: if I thought I had $25 to spare right now—and if that was *all* I had to spare—by what right did it go to Ken Hertz? Why not to the city's hungry, to a women's shelter, to any of a number of worthy charitable organizations—or to research on Parkinson's, for that matter? Why to this one person? To which there was only one possible answer: Ken Hertz had asked. And kept asking.

Then I'd forget about him until he asked again.

In February of 1989, exhausted by the stresses of my life as a single mom and the emotional turmoil involved in ending a 19-year marriage, I stepped off a city bus, bent to retrieve the woolen beret I'd dropped in the slush—and failed to get up again. There was an explosion of pain in my lower back, a sensation as of a cork popping, followed by "fireworks" in my spinal column. The pain when I tried to stand was insupportable. I sank back to the pavement, my legs jumping spasmodically. Passersby called an ambulance, and I was carried into Emergency strapped to a board. This was around 1:30 in the afternoon; in my head, I was still calculating that I could be back from the hospital in time to meet my kids home from school at 4:30. When it became apparent that I might not be (and how was I going to *get* home, anyway?), I had an orderly wheel my bed to the pay phone so I could make arrangements with a neighbor.

The next three months of my life was to be a series of "arrangements with neighbors." Neighbors brought me home and carried me into the house. Though the official diagnosis did not come until I was pretty much back on my feet (the waiting period for a CT scan being several weeks), I had herniated two lumbar discs: the initial prescription, based on symptoms, was two to three weeks of "total bedrest." Exactly how I was to manage this, as a single working mother (my kids were 9 and 11)—with no relatives in town other than my invalid grandparents, and barely enough money to get by on—was left to me.

For the first four days, my "ex" moved back in (a bad idea for everybody); after that, neighbors cooked for us, neighbors came in to make sure the kids got off to school on time each morning, neighbors helped with errands. When home, the kids pitched in on chores to the best of their abilities, and I stayed in bed, doped on pills at first, as much as I could. Doze, wake, doze some more, heating pad . . . the monotony was excruciating. But as soon as I could physically manage it, I began getting up to use the toilet and to bathe, I got up to fetch things for myself when nobody else was around. . . . I began to do whatever I could for myself as I found I could do it. A mistake. The day after my three-week follow-up at the hospital (I'd gone by bus, reluctant to pay for taxis) I collapsed again. By then I'd used up my sick leave and bank of paid sick days, and had to go on disability. But I hadn't learned my lesson: I kept getting up too soon—to attend a school event with one child or the other, to do some small local errand that seemed pressing, to bake for a Jewish holiday— and even though I arranged lifts from door to door or took taxis, even though I took care to avoid being on my feet longer than a few minutes at a time—I'd end up on my back again.

I was frightened. I was making no progress. After several weeks of forced inactivity, on a good day I still could barely walk half a block unsupported; I was a virtual cripple. Would I ever fully recover? Was this going to be chronic? And each time I relapsed, the medical advice was the same: two or three weeks' total bedrest. (In fact, if I could arrange it—they told me kindly—I really ought to spend at least ten days in the hospital, in traction. Somehow the idea didn't appeal; what a relief that I couldn't arrange it.)

My world had shrunk to a room, my bedroom. Friends came for a while, but the "emergency" wore off . . . I was managing . . . people had their own problems, I didn't want to prevail on anyone. I had my piles of books, my giant thermos of tea, my telephone. On sunny days, for the hour of afternoon that the sun came into my downstairs flat, I had the shadows of bare branches projected onto my dusty window, and sometimes the shadows of a pair of squirrels, playing—a graceful dance in silhouette. I thought, This is what I must content myself with, this is my share of the outside world these days: such shadows as project themselves onto my window. Pain still woke me hourly most nights, leaving me too sleepy even to read in the daytime . . . every day felt like a month . . . boredom and loneliness gnawed. I felt sad and seedy in my airless room, depressed by my messy neglected house; my own inactivity revolted me, my jelly-like calves, my sagging thighs.

People brought me literature on back problems, recommended chiropractors and naturopaths, told me about Feldenkreis, urged me to do Tai Chi. Still immobilized after ten weeks, I was ready to pull all stops at once. I saw a Japanese doctor who attached electrodes to my back and buzzed me, then bound one of my feet and sent me home with an unmarked bottle of pills made of ground-up adrenal glands (did he really say that, or did I imagine it?)—pebbly, misshapen pills that looked like animal pellets; my god, I thought, these could be *anything*, and I'm taking them? I saw him again, and he told me to take supplements of zinc and manganese; he told me to have a back scan; he told me Feldenkreis wouldn't do a thing if what I had was a herniated disc. He did some pushing and pulling and I thought I felt a little better, but a few hours later there was something wrong with my left arm and shoulder, in fact now the whole left side of my body was out of commission. I took the zinc and manganese.

I saw the top back surgeon in the city (I had to scream and yell to get an appointment)—a beefy man with a face startlingly devoid of intelligence—who repeated the prescription for bedrest, then said without a trace of humor, "Eighty-five percent of herniated disc patients improve with bedrest after a few weeks. Of course, I make my living off the fifteen percent who don't. . . ." I saw a psychiatrist, who told me to see a neurologist. I saw a neurologist who scratched the soles of my feet, made one of his fingers disappear before my eyes, and ordered a brain scan (which registered normal). I saw a social worker.

In the end, I think, I got better out of sheer will; I galvanized myself back to mobility in a lightning-hot paroxysm of rage at the entire medical system, my own helplessness, the cumulative irritant of everyone's inane remarks and inept suggestions. (The unfortunate target, or conduit, for this bolt of passion was a telephone receptionist in Radiology at the Montreal General who informed me that I could not have possession of my own X-rays.) The day after my outburst, miraculously, I woke up without pain. . . . I got up and walked (a block and a half, in soft spring rain) . . . without pain. I decided I wasn't doing "bedrest" any more. Pain came and went for a while—it came back if I overdid things—but never with the same incapacitating intensity; my legs no longer gave out, my hips had stopped "locking," the stiffness in my upper body was gone. Inexplicably, but unmistakably, I was on the mend.

My ordeal had lasted three months, almost to the day. How quickly it fell behind me as my world expanded outward again! How readily I came to take for granted, as before, the mundane miracle of my own mobility, the truth of the quote from Feldenkreis—"Life is motion"—that I'd copied into my journal. But I did not forget entirely. I knew I'd come close to something fundamental, I had been touched by something.

Months slipped by; a letter came from Ken Hertz. The usual letter. He was still campaigning for fetal-cell surgery. This time, not quite caught up on family expenses after my weeks on disability, I couldn't even spare the paltry $25. But the thought of this man in his forties, his mental faculties intact—housebound, bedridden, paralyzed, sustaining himself on faint hope—tugged at me. I sat down and wrote a short letter. I could send no money for the moment, I explained, but I had not long ago spent three months immobilized by a back injury, and I felt for him: perhaps he would like a visitor.

A few days later the phone rang; a female voice with a Caribbean accent informed me that Ken Hertz was calling. "Ken has received your letter. He says he would like a visit." The speaker, who did not identify herself, gave me instructions on how to get to Ostell Crescent. (It wasn't near, and the transportation from my home was awkward.) We arranged a day and a time; I was to call before coming.

I found Ken Hertz in the small, somewhat shabby front room of a cluttered, untidy upper duplex across from the Jewish cemetery where, six years later, he would be buried. At that time, he had not left his room for three years. (The rented flat was the home of his ex-wife—they had been divorced several years before he fell ill—and her two children from a subsequent relationship; Hertz laughed out loud at the look on my face, or the irony of the situation, when this was explained to me.) His around-the-clock paid helpers—I learned there were six of them, working in shifts—seemed to be mainly West Indian women, impassive and impersonal; they did not introduce themselves to me on the phone or in person. A young girl, a college student, who sat on a futon under the window writing out letters and addressing envelopes by hand, was more communicative.

I don't know whether Hertz remembered me, but I recognized the small, slight figure on the bed—balding, with a narrow face, graying beard, intense eyes behind wire-rimmed lenses—from our one or two passing encounters at launches and literary gatherings. He did, however, know who I was. Eyelids fluttering furiously with the effort, he managed to expel the single sentence: "How is Fred?" And I had to explain we were divorced; our small-press enterprise had folded; I hoped Fred was fine, but couldn't speak for him.

The burden was clearly on me to do most of the talking—an awkward business, given that I didn't really know the person I was talking to. I spoke of my three months on disability, how interminable they had seemed to me, how I marveled at his—Ken's—staying power. I spoke of acquaintances we had in common. I asked questions, which he answered in the affirmative or negative by means of hand or eye signals interpreted for me by his helpers. Sometimes he managed to get out a few words of his own: at this time he was still able to murmur, and occasionally even to speak a full sentence in a startlingly normal voice. His face had the mask-like rigidity typical of Parkinson's, but that was broken frequently by a transfiguring smile, one reflex the disease seemed to have spared him. Every few minutes—confirming the bizarre description in his letters—his attendants would grasp his hands and rock him forward into a sitting position, swing his legs off the bed, stretch his arms, massage his hands and feet, then swing him back again. It happened wordlessly, in an almost dreamlike rhythm; you soon stopped noticing it.

I learned during this visit that Ken's 24-hour care was costing some $8000 a month, of which only $1000 came from the government. (Later a Jewish philanthropic organization kicked in to cover another chunk.) The government, which Hertz had petitioned the previous year to pay his home care costs, would have paid in full for his placement in a chronic-care institute—but Ken was convinced (rightly, according to doctors) that he would not live very long in a hospital setting. He was severely allergic to industrial cleansers. But more importantly, no chronic-care facility could promise to move him every five minutes, around the clock—a treatment he had devised for himself, to which he attributed his continuing stable condition. Doctors had expected

him to succumb years earlier to pneumonia or some other com-
plication of long-term immobility; the team of Mexican doctors
who decided against surgery said that his case of Parkinson's was
the most severe they'd seen. But Ken Hertz chose not to take L-
dopa, a drug that could restore some mobility, on any kind of
regular basis—because of its side effects (acute anxiety, halluci-
nations) and because he believed that each time he took it, he
was left permanently worse after its effects wore off.

I visited Ken infrequently over the next few years—the demands of my own life being complicated, my emotional reserves
low. But it did not take many visits to become familiar with his
strange world. Not much seemed to change in the small room
on Ostell Crescent: the faces of some of the helpers, but not
their routines. One black woman on a chair by the bed, at the
ready, a kind of sentinel; another sitting at the foot of the bed,
maybe crocheting; at five-minute intervals both moving in uni-
son, as if at an internal signal, into the silent dance with the figure on the bed. On the futon, sometimes as many as three young
women writing out letters, collating Xeroxes, stuffing envelopes—silently and diligently churning out the fund-raising
packages that kept Ken alive and out of an institution while he
waited and hoped for "The Operation," the miracle cure. It was,
I saw, a system, a functioning small business—Ken's invention.
The room was full of his inventions. The plastic drinking-straw
with notches cut in it so he could hold it with his teeth. The
pocket full of cards with messages he could point to: JUICE.
PEE. ENEMA. OPEN WINDOW. CLOSE WINDOW. MASSAGE
SHOULDERS. RADIO. TELEPHONE. ALPHABET. MAIL.
BANK—TAKE OUT $. If he pointed to TELEPHONE, there was
a card with people's names and numbers—the speaker-phone
rang frequently as friends and supporters checked in or returned his calls. If he pointed to ALPHABET, there was a card
printed with block letters so Ken could point-spell a message not
otherwise covered. Visitors seemed to float in and out. On the
wall were a few paintings; almost always, the radio was playing
(no TV—Ken told me he didn't like TV); sometimes the tape
deck. When I visited, I usually read aloud—at Ken's request
some of my own poems, or a story in progress—but also other
writers, anything I happened to feel like sharing that day. I never
knew how long to stay; I always felt awkward leaving. But one

thing became clear, and it made me feel a little better about the spacing of my visits: isolation was not one of this man's problems. A shut-in he might be, but Ken Hertz was not languishing alone in his little room; constellations of individuals clustered around him, involved in one way or another in the peculiar web that was his life.

I came to dread his phone calls. First the hollow echoing static of his speaker phone, then the remote female voice: "It's Ken Hertz calling—" (the voice clipped off, swallowed by bad reception at my end). "Yes, hello, can you hear me?" I'd ask stupidly, and wait for the pause, hiss, "Yes, go ahead, we hea—" Bad at one-way conversation face-to-face, I felt hopeless about it on the telephone; I felt put on the spot. What could I say? Should I talk to Ken—who I knew could not answer—or should I address the nameless caller? "How are you, Ken?" I'd ask, and again there'd be that hollow echoing pause, before the same voice came back with the standard reply (it began to seem a macabre joke): "Ken says he's a little stiff today." Always I hoped to hear news—that "The Operation" was imminent (all this while his letters continued to arrive like clockwork, each time implying that a date for the fetal-cell implant would soon be set)—but no, "Ken is still trying to raise the money" or, "We're waiting to hear from the doctor," "We're hoping the hospital will call us soon." Then, with a little trepidation, I'd ask, "Ken, is there any special reason you're calling me?" Long pause; background rustling; echo and hiss. And finally (and oh how chastening, his usual answer)— "No, Ken just wants to say hello."

Was the operation a real possibility, or a pipe dream—was Ken deluding himself? As the date kept getting pushed back (at first, it seemed, because of controversy over the use of fetal cells; later it wasn't clear why)—monies collected toward the surgery repeatedly had to be siphoned off to cover his home care costs. Yet Hertz continued to campaign for funds on two platforms—for ongoing home care, and for the fetal-cell implant in Denver. It was hard to imagine him being able to save toward the one while paying for the other; I thought I could see why the operation kept being deferred.

Others had their own spin on things. One local writer (who, unlike me, had known Ken personally for years before he became ill) told me she thought the real issue was that Ken had a "pathological terror of dying." She questioned his moral right, as an individual—at a time when the homeless and destitute were all around us—to prevail on the help of the public to prolong indefinitely, at great expense, a kind of half-life with no concrete hope of improvement. "I wouldn't ask that," she told me, "You wouldn't ask that. There are others in need—there are sick babies, curable babies, who haven't had their chance at life yet, who could live full lives. Why is this particular life worth more than any other? The operation is a long shot—even if he has it, there's no guarantee it will help him . . . I think his credibility with the public is breaking down . . . friends are distancing themselves. Maybe it's time for Ken to stop resisting his own death. Maybe it's just time for him to die."

Hard as her words sounded, I couldn't deny I'd had similar troubled (and troubling) thoughts. And yet: here was this will. This tenaciousness of a man not to die. The implacable strength of one man's will to stay alive, the absolute conviction that *his life* was "worth it." A man whose parents were dead, whose only brother—estranged, it appeared—was in Hong Kong, a man with no property, no heirs, no visible family but an ex-wife who had extended to him a room in her rented flat; a man who was unable to walk, talk, sit up, or change positions unaided. This was the man who had made an institution, a business, of *not dying*; he had made *not dying* his life—and if the system he had devised to sustain it drew upon public and private money, it also offered paid employment to a number of people. The whole thing was in its way astonishing, confounding, outrageous—and oddly inspiring. It took people strangely. Another woman told me she had made a commitment to send money to Ken on a monthly basis for as long as he remained alive—"the same amount every month. I take the attitude that he is showing me I can afford to spare this money each month . . . right now, it's helping Ken; when he dies, I know it will be able to go to help others."

"Ken is very unusual. Something about him motivates people," said Mary Hagey, one of the Hertz home-care entourage, in an interview with a local weekly in 1991. A literature student who worked for Hertz over a summer, she became intrigued with his history as a poet, researched his writings, and wrote a paper on him that was published in the review, *Matrix*. The same year,

Hertz's youthful poems were published for the first time in book form by his friend Leonard Angel; *The Cracked Cellar* was launched at the Jewish Public Library, in yet another bid to raise funds for surgery. Hagey and others observed that a number of the poems, surreal and death-obsessed, written when Hertz was still a teenager, seemed disquietingly prescient of the fate that would overtake him—almost as if something in his personal psychology predisposed him to the disease, or sensed it incubating in him. It was one more facet of a singular, sometimes disturbing, always surprising story.

I visited Ken again. He looked the same, but he was less able to speak, and the notched drinking straw was gone—he now drank from an infant's bottle. I read to him for an hour, left when another visitor arrived. As I went out, I noticed a memo on the wall by the door: "If Ken falls on the floor, dial 911 but ON NO ACCOUNT LET THEM TAKE HIM TO THE HOSPITAL."

I thought I was beginning to understand. Ken wanted to die at home, if he was going to die. Perhaps on some level the "operation" he was waiting for was his own death. In his last letter he had again referred to an operation that showed "great promise of alleviating" his condition; he'd said, "It is very difficult to wait for the operation." Fetal-cell surgery might, at this juncture, be real, or it might have become a metaphor, a light in the distance (the man was, after all, a poet)—but if a fetal-cell implant was not forthcoming, there was that other "operation" which would free Ken from the prison that his own body had become. The one that, when all's said and done, we're all waiting for.

In March of 1994 *The Gazette*—the Montreal daily that had been covering the Hertz story for over a decade—blew Ken Hertz out of the water. In a front-page story headlined *The Ken Hertz Story. . . . It's Not What It Seems*, staffer Debbie Parkes disclosed that a telephone call to the doctor in Denver (whose name Ken invoked regularly in his fundraising literature) had confirmed that Hertz was not on the waiting list for fetal-cell surgery—"and never had been." Apparently the doctor had met with Hertz years earlier, while in Montreal for a conference, and had explained that to be considered for the procedure, Hertz would first (among other things) have to be on a trial of L-dopa for a six-month period. Hertz had refused the drug regimen. Moreover, the local neurologist Hertz was still naming as his doctor claimed to be a consulting physician only—having not personally treated Hertz for nearly a decade.

The city's three English-language weeklies were unanimous in condemning *The Gazette's* tone and spirit, but the damage was done: the effect of the article was to destroy Ken's fundraising base. Corporations that had regularly sent four-figure checks no longer did. Donations dropped immediately by half, and things went downhill from there. Obliged to accept welfare, Hertz in 1995 came under the care of the Public Curator; his helpers were dismissed and replaced, his condition deteriorated, and on the night of January 28, 1996, dehydrated and infected with mild pneumonia, he was taken to the hospital (apparently against his will) by Urgence Santé. He died a few hours later.

Sad to confess, I had fallen out of contact with Ken in the last couple years of his life, as my own life evolved and knit itself, crowding with new commitments. I sent money—the usual small amounts—when I was able. His phone calls still came now and then, and I responded each time by writing him a letter—the kind of chatty communication I couldn't manage to deliver impromptu on the phone. I wrote to him when the *Gazette* article appeared; I said the presentation was certainly unfortunate, but that I thought Parkes *had* made some good points—about the relatively low cost of home care and the right of a patient like Hertz to be cared for at home (if that was his choice) under government subsidy. I said I hoped that was what thinking readers had gotten out of the article; and I enclosed a larger check than usual, in case they hadn't.

The revelation that Ken Hertz was not slated for fetal-cell surgery did not surprise me; I had been reading between the lines of his communications for years. But something else— something I learned only after his death—did surprise me. Asked by *The Globe and Mail* to write an obituary column on Hertz, I delved into his file box at the Jewish Public Library and came across some fairly recent press clips that I'd missed when they appeared. From them I learned that Ken did occasionally take a form of L-dopa, and that under its effects, even in his last year, he was able for as long as a couple of hours to converse normally, enjoy a take-out meal (which he could eat unaided), and move about—if somewhat clumsily—on his own steam. I felt momentarily hoodwinked—as though something, a crucial piece of a puzzle, had been kept from me. These periodic "mini-awakenings" explained, then, how Ken could instruct and organize the people who worked for him, effectively remaining at the helm of his own affairs. But why was I never told of this? How often did it happen? Clearly, it would not have been in the interests of his campaign for too many people to see him in this state; and it would not have been reasonable to expect Ken, in honor of my visits, to swallow a pill with deleterious side effects just so he could speak to me. Still, it gave me an odd feeling to learn that the drug Ken insisted was not an option for him may, after all, have been a major player in his survival system.

Ken Hertz suffered a debilitating terminal illness for much longer than many would willingly have chosen to endure it. I suffered a mercifully brief (though it felt interminable) temporary debilitation. Rendered physically helpless and dependent, both of us chose to accept or reject medical advice according to our intuitive sense of what we needed to preserve our autonomy: Hertz rejected L-dopa as a regimen, but used it when it served the purposes of his own survival plan; I modified the prescription of "total bedrest" according to tolerance—such movement as I could tolerate physically, such bedrest as I could tolerate morally. Each of us rejected the hospital, that notorious divestor of autonomy—I, though it promised to cure me; he, because he thought it would kill him. In the end, I believe, Hertz died when he lost control of his life—I got better when I seized control of mine.

Why were people willing to keep sending money for an experimental operation—a stab in the dark, a piece of magical thinking, an expensive lottery ticket—but not willing to keep sending it to maintain the personally directed care system that for twelve years sustained a "hopeless" case of Parkinson's, not only keeping the man physically alive but affording him a measure of autonomy, of personal dignity? Why was the government unwilling to pay for such care, when the cost of institutionalized chronic care would have been the same or higher? Did Ken Hertz keep invoking "The Operation" because he needed that hope to keep himself going—or because he was shrewd enough to realize that the public needed that hope, to want to go on helping him? *What is a life we are personally willing to sustain?* These are the kinds of questions Ken's story raises for me. Was the "kindness of strangers" being lavished all those years to keep Hertz alive—or to keep *hope* alive? Or had Hertz the silenced poet, in an act of enormous egoism turned inside-out, somehow made of himself a last poem, a human symbol of hope?

Hertz held a press conference in his room, a week after the *Gazette* article appeared, protesting that the newspaper had subjected him to false accusations and innuendoes in order to undermine his financial support. While he did not provide documentation to support his contention that he was on a waiting list for fetal cell surgery (and *The Gazette* stood by its story), Hertz insisted that *he, and all sufferers of Parkinson's disease, were potential candidates for such an operation.* As long as he had the will and the means to keep himself alive, that was "waiting list" enough for him.

The Hertz story remains, for me, something of an enigma. His life, his death. His strange symbiosis with a public that was pulled into the vortex of his personal will to survive. His existence on the fringe and in the face of the medical system; his implacable endurance, physical and moral. The last time I saw him, when I came to stand by the bed, the rapid tremorous blinking of his eyes made me think of a trapped soul, fluttering to free itself from the grip of his frozen body. But when I touched his swollen twisted hand saying goodbye, I found it warm.

I think back to those three months when my own life collapsed in on itself—when my body ceased to come under the jurisdiction of the mind that tried to animate it—when the basic connections we take so for granted, the *life* connections, broke down in me. I remember those three months: my body become freight, my world reduced to a room. Was I any less alive then, was I any less human, was I any less *myself*? I know that I was not.

REHEARSAL

That night, Aileen insisted we eat dinner at the Q, our favorite downtown restaurant.

"I'll call it a hairball," she said, twisting her fork in fettucine.

"Good God, why?"

"I don't know. I like to think of it as something I can puke out."

"Please, let's take this seriously."

"No," she said, lifting her glass of chardonnay. "I'm thirty-two, don't smoke or work with chemicals. I drink moderately. There's no reason I should have cancer, so for the moment I'd like to think of this as a hoax. Cancer in my colon, sex with aliens, Elvis Presley lives."

She steered her glass toward me, and I responded out of duty. Our first morbid toast. She would, as the few months passed, offer many more. And then she had the morphine, and she didn't need wine any longer.

That night at the Q, I did little more than touch the chardonnay to my lips. I didn't want the taste. I didn't want to smell the smoked salmon on my plate, or to nod politely at the waiter who asked us, "How's everything?"

"Let's play a game," I said. This was a thing with us since before our marriage, playing hypothetical games. "You're trapped on a deserted island, and you can have only one person there, one piece of music, and one book. What do you bring?"

She tapped her fingers against the wine glass, her wedding band ringing the stem. "The book," she said, "is the Bible. For inspiration and entertainment. The music," she said, suddenly sentimental, reaching for my hand and wiggling her fingers through mine, "would be a performance of one of your operas. Maybe *Anna Karenina*. Maybe The *Inferno*. Depends how it turns out. The person, of course, would be you."

"And say you had terminal cancer," I said, feeling not senti-mental but desperate, as if I would yank her across the table into my lap. "Time would be short. What's your fantasy, then?"

She waited as a busboy splashed our water glasses from a clear pitcher swaddled in linen. What he spilled spread in a wide blot, darkening the table cloth. The boy apologized, then moved on.

"Your fantasy?" I said.

"Live as long as I can," she answered. "And die before I can't stand it anymore."

The following Sunday, I woke before dawn to work—rehearsals had started, and I wasn't yet satisfied with the aria I'd composed for Dante to deliver at Hell's Gate—but I couldn't concentrate on the score, so I quit to let Max, our two-year old beagle, take me for a walk. When we got back to our loft, it was time to get ready for my regular Sunday date with Aileen: strong coffee and Vivaldi while dressing, Mass at St. Cyril's, then bagels and the Sunday paper at our favorite bistro. Usually these were festive mornings, but as I brought a mug of coffee to her in bed, she asked that I not put on any music.

"I'm tired of happy sounds," she said, pressing the heels of her hands against her forehead. "All week long, I've listened to peo-ple make happy sounds for my benefit. It's the day of rest. Can we just have quiet?"

"Of course," I said, and I sat beside her, and we stayed that way, sipping our coffee, not speaking, until she set her mug on the end table and closed her eyes.

"Aileen?"

"I'm not going to church," she said. "Not today. I can't today."

"I'll stay home, too."

"No," she said. "I'd like bagels. I'd like you to bring me some bagels on your way home. Will you do that for me?"

I nodded, and she smiled. "You're sweet," she said.

Max came alongside the bed, carrying his bald tennis ball, slapping his tail against the mattress. Aileen took the ball from him and threw it out the door, bouncing it across the hardwood floor of our loft. Max charged after, and I stretched to watch him slide into the walls as if indestructible.

Aileen sighed. Her face acquired a look of distance: a little fur-row of the brow, a slight parting of the lips. She nodded as if in agreement with herself.

"Let's play a game," she said. "Say you're out for a walk with Max, and he bolts across a busy street and gets hit by a truck." She paused as if waiting for my imagination to start.

"I don't like this," I said, suddenly empty and afraid because I knew, somehow, what was coming. I had expected it since that night at the Q when she talked about dying before she couldn't stand it. "We should be past games, now," I said.

"Max survives," she went on, "but the vet says he's lost all mobility. He'll be stuck in his little doggie bed the rest of his life. Might not be a long life anyway."

"Aileen, stop it."

"Also, he's in pain. Please, Reid. He's in pain."

It was the only cruel game she'd ever played. I looked out our window at the vacant, late autumn. Not a bird. Not even a wisp of a cloud. I couldn't breathe. My chest hurt that much.

"Jesus, Aileen. I want to keep you, not help you go. Why are you even thinking about this now?"

She took my hand, pulled it toward her and hugged it against her body.

"Because I'm scared to think about it by myself."

I went to Mass like she asked. What would I otherwise do? Besides, part of me needed church, needed to plead our case to God. I'd tried all week—little bits of why and please, frantic yearnings in the middle of the night aimed at Him—but no true prayers.

My umbrella and overcoat barely sheltered me from the chilly November rain as I neared the church steps, and I slipped climbing the worn, wet marble. I reached for her to anchor me, regained my footing anyway, and walked on, disconsolate. In the dimly-lit foyer I accepted a weekly bulletin from the regular usher, a grandfatherly type who asked, "Where's that good-looking redhead?" "Not feeling well," I said, then blessed myself with a spattering of holy water. Walking into the church, I felt like a stranger, unwelcome, as if I were already dirty with the sin Aileen had asked me to consider.

She and I always sat midway toward the altar. This day, though, I wanted God to notice me.

I passed our usual section, waving to a few acquaintances, then genuflected at the front pew where only the elderly parishioners sat. They nodded and smiled and welcomed my intrusion on their regular company. Kneeling, I clasped my hands and humbled myself with the sign of the cross.

"God," I whispered, "make this go away."

Throughout the service, I prayed: greedy, justifiable prayers, asking that Aileen be made whole, that she be spared, that I be spared. During long meditations, these degenerated into repetitions of "Please, God" and then into flashing visions of my life alone. I saw myself at home, wrecked, composing an opera for her. I pictured myself grieving on Mackinac Island where we had honeymooned, or fleeing to the mountains of central Mexico and meeting a young woman who sold calla lilies and who showed no sadness in her face. But remorse crept in, and I fell back on the Lord's Prayer.

And then I looked up, as if staring Him in the face would convince Him to change the world for me. All I saw were the frescoes tiled like Byzantium, the Ten Commandments in stained glass, the tops of pillars beyond my reach. What on most Sundays inspired me as regal and mysterious, on this morning discouraged me as aloof and haughty.

That was that. I left the service in low spirits, eager to be home. Once there, I kissed the forehead of my napping wife and the bangs across her forehead. She woke at the touch of my lips and smiled and laid her hand around the back of my neck, tugging the small hairs there.

"How's God?"

"Same as always."

"Did you bring bagels?"

I grimaced. "I'll go right away," I said.

"No. Stay now."

She pulled me in. We lay on the couch, and I felt the press of her body as she breathed, the confidence in her arms as she held me, and those things collaborated to restore for me our shining, mundane world. Later, as I napped, she made brownies. We watched basketball together in the afternoon. UConn's women won.

The next week, surgery showed the cancer had metastasized into Aileen's liver and kidneys.

We lived on the third floor of a converted factory where other artists and musicians lived, and they would stop by our loft unbidden, say something heartfelt and Aileen would respond,

"That's kind, thank you. Well, nice of you to stop by," and so the well-wishers began to fall away and not call. Before she had always liked company.

She cut back on her hours at the Wadsworth Gallery, then abruptly quit. We filled her free time with walks when she felt up to it, or with romantic summer-love movies we rented on video. Besides me, the only other person she'd talk to about the cancer was her sister Amy—her only family—whom she would telephone on the West Coast.

Shortly after Aileen's surgery, while taking out the garbage, I ran into Maria-Marie Chapman in the hallway outside our apartment. She carried a poinsettia in a plastic pot wrapped with foil, and she offered it to me. Maria-Marie lived on the fifth floor. She had been a neighbor long before I met Aileen, and Maria-Marie and I had moved beyond neighborliness on a few nights. Now we seldom talked, though we had ample opportunity. She sang soprano with the Hartford Opera Company, which produced most of my work. In the *Inferno* opera, I'd written for her the part of Francesca, condemned for lust to an eternal whirlwind with her lover Paolo. A little joke. Besides, Maria-Marie looks to me how I imagine Francesca: a creamy forehead, violet eyes, and a dark, sorrowful mouth. I accepted the poinsettia; she took our garbage and asked about Aileen.

"She's feisty," I said. "She's decided against chemo or radiation. Says she's too sick to be sick. Pain scares her. Sometimes she watches TV all night to keep from worrying about the pain."

One reason I didn't talk with Maria-Marie anymore was that I always told her too much. Others in my circle had the same problem—the men did, at least. We all told Maria-Marie too much. Immediately I felt a sliver of guilt for revealing the intimacies of my wife's illness to someone who should be a stranger.

Maria-Marie leaned into the sill of one of the hallway's high plexiglass windows, inlaid with wire and scratched opaque from factory days. "I was amazed to see you at rehearsals," she said. "I think I'd just fold up and—oh, just fold up."

"Aileen says I should work. She wants everything to be as it's always been."

"But it's not," she said, as if arguing. "Well, everybody needs some pretense to get by. Tell her I'm thinking about her, will you?"

I said I would, and brought the poinsettia into the apartment, feeling as if that act compounded my little betrayal. Aileen never noticed Maria-Marie's gift—our loft looked like a greenhouse, we had received so much flora—and I never brought it to her attention.

Our car was on the blink, and we couldn't afford to fix it—not with deductibles and co-payments—so I was taking the city bus to rehearsals. The route ran helter-skelter and took a half-hour longer than driving, but the bus did stop at the corner downtown where the opera company had turned a defunct department store into its headquarters.

I stepped off the bus one morning—the same morning we expected the arrival of our principal tenor, the semi-famous Ricardo Furmansky—when I heard a woman's voice sing out my name in B flat major. When I turned I saw Maria-Marie drive past in her car, Furmansky in the seat beside her, a suitcase in his lap. Later I learned they knew each other from performing *La Traviata* in Tulsa. Maria-Marie waved and Furmansky raised a steaming convenience store cup, as if toasting me with his coffee.

We rehearsed in what had once been the toddlers' section of the department store. Pink ponies and cartoon giraffes still smiled at us from the walls. When I arrived, the conductor sat at the piano trying to help a baritone graduate student from Amherst negotiate a few of my bars.

"Leave this transgrrrrresor to meeeee," he sang. We had hired him for a bit-role as one of Lucifer's devils. "Hell-bound he is! For to rrrrepent the sin while sinning is not to rrrrepent at aaaaall."

"No," complained the conductor. "Curb your oscillation. You sound like a goddam bleating sheep." He turned to me. "Good morning, Reid."

I nodded toward him, then took my seat and opened my score. This part of the Inferno, the story of Count Guido da Montefeltro, had always troubled me. It was about sin, of course, but also about human nature. A conniving pope had forced the Count to do evil, bestowing absolution in advance for any sin committed by his command. But that wasn't good enough, even if the Count regretted the sin as he committed it. As one of Dante's devils stole the Count's soul to Hell, he exclaimed that it was impossible to, at the same time, willfully sin and repent the sin. Such cold logic seemed to me inhumane, too black and white for a poet like Dante who understood the colorful complexities of life. I'd written the scene into the opera to try to understand it. Not so some graduate student could turn my work into melodrama.

"I don't like how that sounds," I said. "Let's make the high C a G, and have him sing softer."

He announced the changes to the student, then added, ". . . and resonate. Use your cheekbones."

I hated rehearsals, wasting time in an uncomfortable chair while egos rotated in and out to practice. At home, the laundry stood waist high. The batteries were dead in our television remote control, and I needed to get replacements so Aileen could watch. She needed me to adjust the thermostat and fetch her tapioca. I needed to be with her.

"You have to see it through," she had said. "This is your best piece."

About that, she was right. The music excited me, filled my soul and swept me off—which felt wrong. There were moments—God help me—I forgot about Aileen at home, just lost track. I think she had that in mind. She sent me away, I think, in preparation.

Furmansky and Maria-Marie arrived as we finished with the graduate student. We shook hands, I took my chair, and as Furmansky warmed up, Maria-Marie came and kneeled beside me. She asked why I was riding the bus, and I told her.

"I can bring you to rehearsal," she said. "And I can bring you home. Whatever help you need. We can run errands if you like. Whatever." She shrugged a shoulder, emphasizing again the "whatever."

I hesitated and looked at my score, open across my lap. She tilted her head to better see my face.

"I mean, if Aileen doesn't mind," she said.

Aileen didn't like Maria-Marie. Not because she and I shared a past, however brief and noncommittal. That was no threat. Aileen disliked Maria-Marie because she considered her superficial and an exhibitionist, especially after her insistence on being listed only as *Maria-Marie* in playbills and programs. Still, I needed help. It seemed rude to say no.

Maria-Marie drove me home after rehearsal that day.

"I love the *Inferno*," she said as we walked the garbage-strewn block to the parking garage where she'd left her car. "It's so gruesome. Decapitations. Flayings. It makes great opera. All the sin."

"That's why I wanted to compose from it," I said. "I'm fascinated by sin."

"What opera fan isn't?"

"But it's the punishment, too. Blasphemers scorched by burning rain. Hypocrites bearing the weight of leaden robes. Punishment completes the sin and satisfies the sinner. Otherwise it's just random, animal violence."

"You think about this a lot?"

"Too much."

She unlocked the passenger-side door, and I reached across to let her in. When she started the car, her CD player powered up in the middle of Mimi's first act aria from *La Bohème*. She turned it off and, as we drove out of the garage, asked me to change the prosody of one of her lines.

"It would work better," she said. "'The shudder of his lips' should shudder, right? I think you want to stretch that over more syllables."

It was a good suggestion, and I agreed to it. She pressed a button and brought back *La Bohème*, then lowered the volume. Neither of us spoke until we were out of downtown and entering the warehouse district.

"Tell me what you've done that's so wicked," she said. "Tell me how you've transgressed that you think about sin too much."

"Maybe it's not what I've done, but what I'm afraid I might do," I said, thinking for a moment about Aileen and Max and games that weren't really games.

"Tell me some past sin anyway."

I shook my head. I don't share my sins, not even with Maria-Marie with whom I share too much. Instead, I hoard them until they boil out of me late at night when I'm supposed to be asleep. This happens now and then. Not often. But when it does, I shiver, I sweat, and my stomach churns as if I've been grazing on remorse since breakfast. I kick away the quilt and feel I'm an acute disappointment—to whom? God?—as I recount my failures and betrayals, however inconsequential. Like the poinsettia.

This is unreasonable, I know, to be so overwrought over something so insignificant. But reason only works for me in the daylight, and then I'm only smart enough to doubt Heaven. Meanwhile, my medieval, superstitious heart still believes—with terrifying certainty—in Hell. Dante's or any other.

I started to attend weekday church services, seeking whatever guidance God might bestow as Aileen grew more ill and suffered greater pain. Maria-Marie met me in our building's lobby at quarter to six each cold morning, then drove me to St. Cyril's. While I prayed with the elderly near the front, Maria-Marie would sit in the last pew, sipping herbal tea from an insulated cup and reading the daily paper. After church, we'd go to rehearsal. Sometimes after rehearsal, we'd run errands.

"How can you stand to be stuck in a car with her?" Aileen asked me. "She's shallow as her purple contacts."

"That's not fair," I said. "She's doing us a favor."

Aileen threw me a look that said, "You're not so stupid as you're pretending."

"If she's making a play for me," I said, "then she'll be disappointed and we'll have had—I'll have had—some help. If she's just being nice, then everything's OK."

Maria-Marie never did come to our apartment. She picked up prescriptions, dropped off laundry at the cleaners, made grocery runs. She listened to my blather. Each morning in the lobby, she would smile and ask how the night had passed. Often, I'd still be talking when we walked into St. Cyril's. "Her sister keeps asking to come, but Aileen's putting it off," I would say, "as if she isn't really sick." Or, shaking my head, "We played Scrabble and she actually used 'tumor' on a double-word score." Or, "I'm so tired of bleaching blood from our sheets."

Sometimes as we drove, if I seemed particularly sullen, Maria-Marie would quietly sing part of her role. At the end she would click her tongue and say, "That's No. 1 this week on Hell's hit parade."

On Christmas day, Aileen couldn't get out of bed. She couldn't eat, and she doubled up every few minutes from the pain.

"Maybe it's menstrual," she said, which we both knew to be a lie. "Turn on the TV for me, will you?"

She watched sentimental Christmas specials, suffered goose bumps, and after one show wept until Max started to howl in sympathy. I poured us a sober man's egg nog to toast the holiday, but she didn't touch hers. When Amy phoned to wish her a Merry Christmas, Aileen asked her to visit soon.

The next day I called a cab to take us to the hospital. They said it was a bowel obstruction. She spent four days away from home, between surgery and recuperation, and on the eve of her release swore she would not go back. "Everything's so white it makes me think I'm dead," she said. "Once I'm home, I want to stay. You, me, and Max."

Amy's flight arrived near midnight on a brisk, snow-bright Saturday, and we waited up for her, Aileen drinking fruit punch in the kitchen, me waiting for the headlights of her rental car in our building's parking lot. I enjoy Amy. She likes to touch people—a hand on the shoulder, an arm around the waist—always with the proper timing and never intrusively. She's comforting that way. Maybe you learn that when you've raised five kids. She's also as evangelical as lay Catholics get, with statues of Jesus and Mary in her front yard, and framed embroideries of Bible verses scattered around her house.

Amy would, I knew, want to go to Mass. She would take me every day, and to rehearsals after that. Amy would work overtime to make our lives easier by her visit.

Snow crackled beneath the tires of her car as she pulled into the lot. We hugged when she stepped out, and I carried her luggage, which was only two pieces. She planned a short stay, knowing she would be back.

"Aileen says you're working on some big new show about sin," she said as the elevator doors slid shut.

"A trip through Hell," I said. "It premieres Friday."

"Oh," she said. "I'm sorry I'll miss it."

The next morning—Sunday morning—while Amy and Aileen worked on breakfast, I phoned Maria-Marie and got her answering machine. I told it—told Maria-Marie—that Aileen's sister had arrived, and she had a car, and so she needn't put herself out on our account any longer. I thanked her.

We three went to church that morning; Aileen could never disappoint her sister. It was in all ways a normal service—we even sat in the pews halfway to the altar—except that Aileen spent more time praying than usual, and when she sang hymns she sang louder than usual. As we left with the crowd, the pipe organ sounding "Now thank we all our God," she walked close beside me, an arm tight around my back. Outside, she began to cry. She sat suddenly on the snowy steps, red around her nose and her eyes wet, her mouth pursed until she managed a gloomy smile. I held her. Amy mined for a tissue in her handbag.

"Let's play a game," Aileen whispered to me. "Say that church makes you really sad."

"Then I stay home."

She nodded. For the rest of the week, Amy and I went to morning Mass ourselves. Each day I came away from the service without an answer and without hope. When Amy left Friday afternoon I stopped going to church, too.

Opening night.

In the apartment, the phone rings with wishes of good luck. It rings again. Max slides into the wall and the balding tennis ball escapes beneath the radiator. Aileen scrubs her face. Dabs rouge, then calls me into the bathroom to look because it's been so long since she's worn mascara. Outside our windows, snow slashes this way, then that. We dress. A tux for me. A black satin gown for her with a silk blouse underneath to ward off any chill. The phone rings again. I eat some chalky antacid pills. She swallows enough codeine to get her through the night. I spit shine my shoes. She notices that she's lost weight in her feet. Her pumps are too loose, so she stuffs them with Kleenex. We toast with chardonnay. She takes from the refrigerator an unexpected boutonniere and pins it to my lapel, then leaves her hand over my heart, smiling. The doorbell rings, and Mr. and Mrs. Brower—she's on the company's board of directors—whisk us to the Bushnell Theater and my big moment.

The notices from that night yellow away in a scrap album somewhere. They were better than average, though I can't remember the performance. Mostly, I remember Aileen in that gown, with her hair in a loose bun, tiny curls dangling near her temples, her face showing the air of permanence you see only in those who are free of all distraction, of all dissatisfaction. She kissed me as the performance started, then slipped the long, white glove from her right hand to hold mine. I remember, during the first intermission, after the pagans and the carnal, the gluttons and the heretics, Aileen leaned into me and said, "It's scarier than I thought."

We hurried backstage as the performers took their bows. I met the conductor when he came off, and we embraced. I hugged

Furmansky, and the other tenor who was Virgil. I hugged the set designer and the bass who was Charon, and cheek-pecked the mezzo soprano who was a whore, and when Francesca the lusty sinner appeared in my arms and tried to kiss me I turned my face aside and let her loose.

"Maria-Marie," I said with as much finality as I could muster, "I'm grateful."

And then some bit-part devil tapped my shoulder, seeking an embrace, to which I turned with great regret and great relief.

We rode home with the Browers who were glad to leave early.

That night was the last good night.

The next morning, Aileen stayed in bed until noon, as if her goal had been to attend the opening with all the vitality she could muster, and now she was done. She ate little. Over the next few weeks, she lost more weight. Her skin became sallow and dry and so sensitive she didn't like to be touched. She stayed in her pajamas until they needed to be laundered. She watched television endlessly. Once a week, she gathered enough strength to take a short walk with me and Max. We would call a cab and the three of us would pile in, and the cabbie would take us downtown to Bushnell Park. We went on sunny days, so she could see the light glint off the golden dome of the state capitol. She liked to sit near the park's carousel building—even though it was closed until the spring thaw—and read the graffiti spray-painted over it.

"*Whiz.*"

"*T-Babe.*"

"*My whorz.*"

"Love poetry," she said, "of a sort."

She had her arms wrapped around her as though she were in a strait jacket.

"Remember that game?" she said. "The one about Max?"

I started to shift my feet forward and back, grinding ruts with my boot heels in the crusty snow. I wished the scraping were louder. I nodded.

"I wonder what you think. I wonder what you'd do. I'm not trying to hurt you," she said, scratching Max behind the ears. "But if I weren't around, and Max was in a bad way, I'd want you to put him to sleep. Out of love."

"I'd put him to sleep," I said. "But Max isn't you."

"No," she said. "You love me more."

Amy returned the next week, this time with four pieces of luggage and a return ticket with no date. When she got in she sat beside Aileen and told her she looked good, which was a lie. Later, while Aileen slept, she told me I looked terrible, which was true. The skin around my eyes was loose and dark. I had chewed my fingernails for the first time since adolescence. Rarely did I shave. Before the day at the carousel, I had thought I could do anything for Aileen. I had thought I loved her that much.

"I haven't slept too well," I told Amy.

"Well, go nap then. And shower, too," she said. "Does Aileen no good to see you like this."

I was glad to have Amy back. On the bad days, our loft was too quiet. I had missed the sound of someone in other rooms.

I contacted a local hospice agency that helped prepare our apartment. We rented a hospital bed and medical equipment. Amy and I learned to monitor symptoms, to administer an IV through a catheter, to change bedpans and dressings, and to give painkillers by injection. After the hospice people left, Amy busied herself with laundry. I gave Aileen a sponge bath.

"It'll hurt," she said, frowning.

"I'll be gentle."

I started with her face, dabbing her forehead and cheeks with a soapy sponge, then wiping with a wet cloth. After each spot I washed, I patted her dry. The wiping caused her the most discomfort; she clenched her jaw and sometimes shivered.

"I'm sorry," I said.

She looked away from me as I unbuttoned her pajama top. I spread the folds to either side, exposing her breasts and her abdomen, which was distended and alien. I gulped from a glass of water, gaining my composure, taking a deep breath before I began washing her. When I touched her abdomen she jolted upright from pain and said, "Don't!"

Her hair felt so awful as I stroked it—like fishing line—but she cried and the crying seemed to relax her. When her pain subsided, I buttoned her top, then unsnapped the bottoms.

"Reid, please," she said, reaching out and taking my wrist. "Please. Let Amy."

Her breath came in soggy, rapid and regular puffs. Her lips were wet with tears and perspiration. "Hey, c'mon," I whispered, my voice breaking. "It's all right. It's all right. We'll make it a game. OK? We'll play doctor."

She frowned, snapping her pajama bottoms and mewing some noise that sounded disgusted and angry. She waved me away.

Aileen's pain had advanced beyond teeth gritting, beyond teeth gritting with codeine, and was now at teeth gritting and asking for short injections of morphine. She required distractions. Sometimes the three of us watched movies or listened to music, or I read to them from Thurber and DeVries. Aileen never mentioned again her hypothetical game about Max or our talk by the carousel, except maybe one morning, when Amy was off buying groceries, Aileen took my hand and sobbed, "I'm sorry," over and over.

The Browers loaned me a little money, and we fixed the car. Amy returned her rental, which she had been using to run errands and attend morning Mass at least three times a week. She kept going in our car. "To keep my humanity," she said. After each service, she would mention how it disturbed her that I stayed away.

"For Lent," I said, "I've given up prayer."

"That's too bad," she said. "But you still need to shake some hands, sing some songs. That's all. Go just once."

The next morning at St. Cyril's, I held the door for an elderly couple, then followed them as far as the sanctuary. They continued down the aisle, but I genuflected at the backmost pew in the darkest part of the church. I did not belong with the others, despite what Amy thought. My wife was dying, and I was dying, too. In the *Inferno* and in my opera, when Francesca speaks with Dante, Paolo weeping at her side, she tells him, "Love gifted us with one death" and it is true she and Paolo died simultaneously. But even if they hadn't, even if Paolo had survived, he would have died. Love, I've discovered, always gives lovers one death. One is all it takes.

Aileen's death would kill us. How could I take part in that? Killing our love felt as sinful as killing my wife.

So in the back pew, I asked God to forgive us our death. I prayed with such sorrow and ferocity that I missed the Mass, raising my head only when a few people shuffled by to leave. I mouthed "Amen," crossed myself and stood. But much of the sparse congregation remained—the older folk mostly, including the couple for whom I had held the door. A deacon extinguished the candles, closed the gold-covered Gospel, locked the Eucharist back in the Tabernacle. And when he finished, as if on cue, a woman in the front pew began to speak, her voice reverberating against the vaulted ceilings, "Hail Mary, full of grace, the Lord is with thee."

And then the others joined her: "Blessed art thou amongst women. . . ."

They began a rosary. The voices droned, investing in the words no spirit at all, no pomp. But something in their rhythm reached me, some force swayed my bones. I realized I was the only person not kneeling, so I knelt, and I began to recite with these voices, dry and old as sand. Yet as I matched their words, as my tongue traced the same patterns of pronunciation, I began to feel a communion with perseverance, with endurance, with a sense of shared order. "Pray for us sinners," we petitioned, "now and to the hour of our deaths." Then we began again. And again. And what they did, these old people and their beads, was to assure me of a world everlasting—in spite of union, partition, days of drizzle and days of sun, with Aileen or without. Those left would carry on from the front pew. Those left would carry on. It was the saddest thing.

Aileen didn't look like Aileen anymore. Her cheek bones were like door knobs. She worked her lips with her teeth, and the lips peeled and scabbed. Her hair spread across the pillow like frayed copper wire. And in the middle of her withering face, her irises shined bright indigo—more vital than ever—but that was the morphine shrinking her pupils to pinholes. It was a false sign of life.

"Open the window," she said. "I hear a crowd."

"That's traffic on the highway," I said.

"Where's Reid?"

"Right here." I touched her shoulder.

"Why won't they be quiet? I just want to sleep."

I measured the dose, gave her a shot. In her sleep, she breathed as if afraid, then so shallow I couldn't be sure of it. I put my fingers near her mouth.

On the TV was an old film in black and white. Color made her dizzy. The film was one I didn't care for, so I turned it off and went to where the shades were drawn against the daylight. We'd made it to March, and it was a warm one. Forsythia already bloomed. Even the daffodils took the dare. To me, it seemed remarkable that spring came at all.

Amy came and sat beside the bed. "Take a break, Reid," she said. "It's a beautiful day. Take Max for a walk. I'll sit with Aileen."

Max leapt at my hands when I showed him his leash, his body twisting like an acrobat's, his wagging tail yanking his legs from under him. He strained down the hall and outside the building, clawing the linoleum, gagging himself in hopes of a good run.

I set him loose at the park nearest our building, a much duller park than the one downtown. No carousel. No golden domes. Just a field of pale, trampled grass no better than dirt, broken by an occasional ghost of a tree. A park Aileen detested as sterile, near death. Still, Max lunged about, oblivious to Aileen's tastes, a black and brown bantam, stripped of everything but speed and a desire for speed. Watching him made me cry.

Afterward, I couldn't return to our apartment right away. I wanted to talk with someone, anyone about anything. The weather. The Red Sox. Specials at the grocery store. In the building's elevator, I pressed the button for the fifth floor.

Maria-Marie answered my knock. Her hair was held back by a kerchief, and she wore yellow scrubbing gloves and blue jeans that were soaked around the knees. Her eyes were a dull gray, a color I didn't recognize as part of her face.

"Reid," she said. "How's Aileen?"

I shook my head.

"She's resting. Her sister is with her." I glanced down at Max. "I just took the dog for a walk. Thought maybe I would say hello."

She invited me in. I sat on her couch, Max resting at my feet, all the run gone out of him. She brought me a cup of herbal tea. Then she sat next to me, tucked her legs beneath her. Pulled off her kerchief.

"Tell me about your day," I said.

She looked around the room. "I did the windows, mothballed the winter clothes." She turned to me, breathed, and smiled a small, failed smile. "I haven't seen you for so long. I hoped you wouldn't look so sad," she said. She reached for my hands, entwined her fingers amidst mine.

"You do look so sad," she said.

I felt my jaw lock, then shudder a bit. I closed my eyes.

"Don't cry," she whispered. "Don't."

She leaned toward me. She was stouter than Aileen, but I was not surprised. I remembered the curve of Maria-Marie's back, and when our foreheads touched I seemed to recall how that felt, too, and the feeling cracked me open, helpless and wanting.

I did not plan that afternoon to break faith with Aileen. I did not plan for what happened next. Maria-Marie touched her fingertips to my cheek, curled them toward my mouth. I kissed the fingers, the knuckles. I opened my arms and let her lean close to me, and she kissed my neck. I needed consolation. I took no time to decide, even though I knew, as I unbuttoned her jeans, that Aileen was downstairs, Amy by her bedside. Maria-Marie's eyes were closed, but I kept mine open because I did not want to think for even a moment that this arm, this bend of hip, this rise of breast, belonged to my wife. The couch was blue felt. On the coffee table sat a half-finished crossword puzzle from the morning paper. I knew what I was doing. I was letting Maria-Marie guide and shelter me. My love-making was clumsy and direct and self-serving. I felt stained, guilty and contrite—but also gifted with a great easing of things, as if by touch of skin and taste of mouth I laid aside old burdens and readied myself for fresh ones. I clenched my fists and whispered an apology.

"It's all right," she said. "Shhhh. It's all right."

I told Amy that Max had caught sight of a cat and given chase, and the next thing I knew we were all the way to Barry Square. That's what took so long. Amy gave me the report: Aileen woke once, my name welling up out of her, then Amy delivered an injection and Aileen relaxed for about five minutes before falling asleep again.

"That seems to be what we get now," Amy sighed. "Delirium or sleep."

"I'll stay with her," I said. "Maybe you should nap."

She nodded. "Wake me in an hour, would you?"

I listened to Amy in the bathroom, heard the toilet flush, heard her brush her teeth and then shut the door to the guest room. I took my wife's hand. She didn't stir. The morphine.

It was near dark and had started to drizzle. Cars floated past on the highway outside, their headlights splintering through the rain that sheeted our windows. I tried to pray, but I couldn't. I thought instead of churches, and I remembered the first wedding I ever attended: an older cousin of mine to a neighborhood girl. I assisted the priest as altar boy. Maybe I was nine. I remember the church was not too crowded, so every cough, every scuffing footfall echoed. My cousin wore curly sideburns and his long hair fell past his powder-blue shirt collar; the bride wore white, carried a bouquet of mums, and she had braces on her teeth. All through the ceremony the best man kept winking at me, nodding toward the betrothed, and grinning as if he and I shared some funny secret. Then the newlyweds kissed, the priest presented them, and they walked, hugging each other and tittering, accompanied by the clapping of family and friends, down the long, red-carpeted aisle toward the huge open doors. The organ rumbled merrily. And I remembered watching the two of them grow smaller, hurrying down the aisle, the two of them alone and shrinking. Later, the best man gave me ten dollars.

My cousin's wife had a daughter five months after the wedding. They've had two more since. My cousin and his wife have been married for so long their oldest is a high school graduate.

Aileen and I were not yet bored with our wedding pictures.

What's right? What's wrong? How do you tell the difference when the sin and the good touch inside you like lovers?

I held my wife's hand. I still wanted the miracle. But with Maria-Marie, I had practiced for the wrong I needed to do and would forever regret. I caressed Aileen's arm, traced my finger over the long vein there. I was weeping.

I would play Aileen's game, the way she wanted me to play.

F. D. REEVE

RELATIVELY DISABLED

Then Clement, the cobbler, cast off his cloak,
And offered it for barter at the game of New Fair.

Then Hick, the horse-dealer, wanting to swap his hood, which was worth less than the cloak, offered his hood and a forfeit in a cap—put his "hand in the cap." He and Clement picked an umpire, who decided the "boot," the size of the forfeit that made the exchange equal. Thus, with the odds set, they finished the sport of the exchange, and in Langland's *The Vision of Piers Plowman* we have the first episode of handicapping in English literature. From the fourteenth-century tavern-lottery to the twentieth-century notion of physical hindrance, handicap odds have been socially defined.

"Handicapped," "disabled," "challenged." Any term we use to describe people whose bodies and minds do not conform to an expected norm quickly becomes pejorative, as "discrimination"—drawing fine distinctions between superficially similar ideas or things—takes a socio-psychological twist and becomes "discrimination"—the assumption that people excluded from one's own group can be defined in terms of group identity without reference to individual merit. Of course, it's hardly news that the handicapped/disabled/challenged, in addition to suffering the physical hassles that accompany living in a society designed for others' needs, have to struggle with discrimination that sees their disability as the sum total of their individuality. But my own experience in the past three years has led me to understand an aspect of this discrimination that receives little press: a disabled person's relatives and close friends are associated in their loss of personal identity.

Because we recognize the roles we play in other people's lives—father, son, husband, friend—as only part of our individ-

256

ual makeup, we welcome them, but when any role becomes all-
encompassing, our individuality—even our sense of self—suffers,
and we "burn out." This happens repeatedly among the disabled
and those close to them.

I learned my place as a "disabled relative" almost immediately
after Christopher, my blue-suited Superman son, broke his neck
at the end of May, 1995. Within days, people—not merely neighbors but casual acquaintances and total strangers—began coming up to me to ask about his health. I soon learned that while
these people's sympathy with Christopher's plight was often sincere, they didn't want to know about his personal, day-after-day
suffering—how precarious his life was, how his health fluctuated,
how close he came to death in the hospital and has come afterward as well. They wanted to hear about his televised role as sufferer—his fight against unconquerable odds—and I, important
to them only as "Superman's Father," was expected to assure
them that the fight was still going on.

The passage of three years has not dulled their enthusiasm:
the more Christopher appears on television, the more frequently
they approach, assuming that I can give them some bit of inside
information that will bring them into the exalted family circle. If
I so much as touch upon the realities of Christopher's situation,
they look puzzled—even betrayed. So I have learned to give
them a "hot tip" on the date of his next important TV appearance, and they leave, somehow assured that by seeing me they
are involved in the good fight and are cheering the underdog.
For me, it's an unrewarding charade, made all the more painful
by the realities of the situation. People who support the "good
fight" have no idea how they're discriminating against—that is,
denying individual identity to—an individual father and son
struggling to maintain a difficult relationship in the face of dif-
fering values and overwhelming physical problems. In Christopher's case, the role of "handicapped Superman" has taken the
place of reality. If I refuse to be de-individualized, or if I insist on
mentioning the misery and hardship that my son feels daily—he
who can never be alone, who must be wakened and turned every
couple of hours during the night—I become a nay-sayer to the
image of which he has become custodian.

The thing Christopher's fans find hardest to believe about me
is that I don't watch television, that in our house we didn't even
have a TV until kind neighbors, concerned that we couldn't

watch Christopher's performances, gave us their old set when they got a big, new one. We keep it upstairs in the guest room closet. When we roll it out to watch a movie, we attach it to a VCR and a closed captioner, which we need because my wife is deaf.

Very interesting is the contrast between being the father of a celebrity with a broken neck and the husband of a deaf novelist-professor. I've learned that while people will go out of their way to help a person in a wheelchair, they assume that someone they can't talk to is stupid, perhaps retarded, definitely to be avoided. The irony underlying the social conviction that the deaf are wit-less goes back to Boccaccio's marvelous story about Masetto, the gardener, who pretends to be deaf to get a job. The nuns believe that because he's deaf he can't be a whole man. Instead of his playing with the girls, the girls play with him. It all ends happily-ever-after "many little monks and nuns" later, but the story does express the popular prejudice that deaf people are dumb. It's a prejudice that holds even among the disabled, as a little sign that used to lie on Christopher's kitchen counter said: IT'S A WHEELCHAIR, NOT A HEARING AID.

At first I was incredulous when Laura said that's how it is, but after many times of witnessing people coldly leaving her out of the conversation—even at the faculty lunch tables in her own col-lege—I admit it's true. Perhaps even more interesting is that peo-ple who talk to me when I meet them by myself cut me out, too, when she and I are together. We try to involve ourselves with them—Laura, a late-deafened adult, speaks clearly and very intelli-gently, and she invariably carries a pencil and pad for communica-tions breakdowns. Sometimes she can read their lips. Sometimes I sign a little for her. But always, after a few minutes, the others turn away and take up with the rest of the group as if we were invisible.

The most stunning instance of our invisibility occurred on a New York street in summer waiting our turn with a group outside a restaurant. My daughter, a research psychiatrist, was there. So was the neurologist who chaired her university hospital depart-ment. He started talking to Laura, but the street shadows were too deep for her to read his lips or to catch any signs. Our daughter explained sympathetically, "She's deaf," whereupon the eminent doctor turned away and spoke to neither of us—even inside at the table—the rest of the evening. If doctors exhibit such discrimination, what can we ask of most people? In fact, what kind of care can we expect or what sort of medical research can we hope for?

Discrimination forces most handicapped people to live peripheral lives, kept out of sight despite their desire to remain a vital part of society. Even a quadriplegic, who knows he can no longer do what he once did, doesn't think himself "handicapped" until society tells him he is. Wisest in many ways are those non-Western societies like the Navajo, which hold elaborate, difficult, imaginative rituals for restoring the deviant spirit to its longed-for social harmony. One of Christopher's significant accomplishments through his many public appearances has been general acceptance of people in wheelchairs. New York is in general a kinder, gentler place, but you also get the feeling that its "kneeling buses" now willingly wait to board wheelchair passengers. To embrace a wheelchair as a fact of life is a huge step forward both in an individual's and in a society's worldly development. Perhaps some day the deaf will be similarly embraced, and my wife and I will be able to watch Christopher's movies in a theater.

Just as there is no beneficent drug which doesn't have undesirable side effects, however, so there is no injury or illness the treatment of which doesn't entail further harm. Some of these side effects have to be harbored by the patient—Christopher has repeatedly suffered dysreflexia, pneumonia, and infection (which kill more quads than the injury does), and when his nurses dropped him, his arm broke. Other side effects, however, have to be borne by those closest to him, his caregivers, whose lives become subordinated to his needs. Once the roles of giving and receiving care become the sum of the relationship between two people, the relationship becomes intolerable. A quadriplegic we know, who doesn't have Christopher's money and must be attended by volunteer friends, had the love of his life break up after eighteen months. Another must be tended by her husband, knowing that he has been forced to change careers in order to keep her alive. Almost all marriages between hearing people quickly end when one of them goes deaf.

Because the disabled can't be whole, whoever voluntarily cares for the disabled can't be a whole person either. Those who contract their services, like any business person, fill partial, eight-hour roles. All of Christopher's two or three dozen attendants—nurses, therapists, drivers and secretaries—are just such professionals, save one—his wife. The professionals move on or off stage according to a schedule, but she can't. Some version of the set figure, or the stereotyped "patient" to whom the professionals minister, gradually comes to dominate for the volunteer the once-beloved individual. Inevitably, the image that serves as a convenience for strangers becomes a projection for the disabled volunteer's psychological relief. Deaf novelist-professor, fallen Superman—it doesn't matter what the disability is.

Public stereotyping of the deaf is no less discriminatory than that of the fallen Superman. Each allows people to sympathize without thinking. Everything in American media encourages people to opt for this sort of response. The difference between admiring a deaf professor's "courage" or a Superman's "good fight" and developing flexible, compassionate understanding of L. Stevenson or of C. Reeve is *thought.*

That said, it's easier to stereotype than to maintain a minute-by-minute consciousness of the interplay of complex personalities in demanding situations. In fact, no one can sustain complex awareness of psychological nuance on a minute-by-minute basis: it's emotionally impossible. Literary and dramatic works at their finest express the subtle acumen of intense consciousness, but they also present stereotypes, for not even the finest novelists and playwrights can develop all their characters simultaneously. Similarly, those who give care—parents and spouses included—have to think in stereotypes some of the time.

The "Fallen Superman" stereotype gives Christopher enormous leverage in his appeals to Congress and on behalf of the American Paralysis Association. For him, and all disabled people, however, the difficulties turn around the ways in which giving and receiving care affect them and their families as well as the ways in which "caregiving" is different from "caring for." Family caregivers not only disappear as individuals in relation to the disabled person but become ancillaries to an image. The late Jean-Dominique Bauby, completely paralyzed except for his left eyelid, superbly handled this irony in his poetic memoir *Le papillon et le scafandre (The Butterfly and the Diving Bell)* by leaping in his imagination out of his body into a different sort of time beyond the reach of all caregiving. There he was free and independent. From there he introduced into his autobiography a precision both of perception and of memory and that element of distancing, or "making strange," by which the power of emotion takes on a life of its own and which distinguishes any genuine literary work.

Too much care infantilizes disabled patients, making them babies by treating them like babies, but it also disables caregivers by wiping out their multiple selves. The closer care*giving* and caring *for* become associated in one person, the more the "good fight" hurts everyone engaged in it. The destructiveness to the individuality is insidious and, like goatweed, wraps itself around the roots of everything: a recent *New York Times* review of Dana Reeve's leading role in *Good Will*, an Off-Broadway play, praised her talent and the believability of her role but defined her as "best known as the wife of Christopher Reeve." Even as an actor, she is confined to one major role; for all her TV and stage appearances, she is as threatened with personal invisibility as I am when I attend a party with my wife.

Compared to the birds of the air and the fish of the sea, we who can neither fly high nor dive deep are all relatively disabled, but we compensate for our disabilities by using machines. At the same time, artistic vision depends on maintaining individuality. The painter Chuck Close, disabled by a stroke, points up the ironic combination of these facts when he says that he can continue as an artist because he can afford the necessary therapeutic machines.

Both the care-giver and the care-taker need worlds of their own in which to reject the stereotyping daily life thrusts upon them and to avoid the terrible temptation offered by the cult of personality—that is, using private grief for public ends like the well-intentioned citizen at the county fair who stopped me, saying, "Mr. Reeve, we'd sure like to take your picture here, playing bingo for the disabled." A cool view of oneself, like a sturdy sense of humor, is necessary to keep the recipient of caregiving from being further disabled by the need for care and the giver of care from becoming a recipient. The limit is marked by one's responsibility for oneself. As old Chinese ethics held that giving alms was immoral because it destroyed a beggar's self-reliance and, therefore, his humanity, so we must look to what preserves our integrity. In whatever self-reliance we're capable of lie our individuality and our worth. How humble and how noble was blind Tiresias, whose insight pierced the ignorance of prejudice and groupthink to illuminate that true discrimination which asserts the individuality of all humans and recognizes their separate dignities in suffering, perception, and merit.

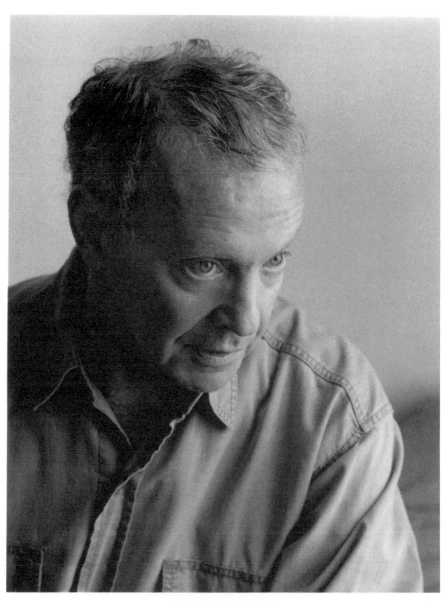

JOSEPH CHAIKIN
Photo: Keith Piaseczny

ECLIPSE

A Theater Workshop on Disability
or, Reflections on Ahab's Tribe

A ragtag Chorus Line confronts a small audience in the New
York Public Theater—an apparently normal couple, two men
with something odd about their gait, a one-legged woman on
crutches, and a man and a woman using wheelchairs. One after
another, and rapid-fire, they ask:

> "Isn't that a tragedy! Can't you sue?"
> "When you go to heaven, will your leg be waiting for you?"
> "Are you more sensitive now with your hands?"
> "If you really wanted to walk, don't you think you could?"
> "Do you cry when you go to the ballet?"
> "Do you still get erections? Can you come?"

This was Joe Chaikin's workshop on disability. The nondisabled
public laughed uneasily. They were hearing questions they themselves might have asked to cover their confusion on encounter-
ing persons with disabilities.

No chronicle of a theatrical triumph, what follows is a memoir
of my participation in an experimental project at a critical moment in my life. For reasons beyond our control, our explorations were cut short and the project remains stalled. Yet facing
and imagining with creative performers what it means to be disabled in our time and place was indispensable to me personally.

It began in the spring of 1994, almost ten years after the stroke
that had left Joe with aphasia at forty-eight, at the peak of his extraordinary career in the theater. In this decade, he had moved
from gibberish to occasional real sentences, though word order
was often scrambled and vowels got lost. We were having dinner
and, given his necessary terseness and abrupt fatigue, running

quickly through the repertoire of topics we'd found intelligible. Joe was telling me that the Public Theater had awarded him a grant, the third in as many summers, to support a two-week workshop of his Disability Project. (His moving battle with despair over his aphasia and his search for means to articulate the experience had become the subject of a handful of plays.) When I learned he was working with actors who were lame, legless, and paraplegic, my interest quickened, as polio had made me limp.

"Who will be your writer this year?"

"Don't know," Joe said.

"Do you want a writer who's disabled himself?"

"Better," he replied in his efficient tongue.

"So, you need me!" I said, "I'm a writer and I'm . . . disabled." And I laughed, because I'd not given it a moment's thought, was just fleshing out the syllogism, and because the word *disabled* felt odd, even phony, applied to myself.

Joe didn't laugh. His mouth made a surprised O, but he said nothing.

Weeks later, he phoned. "Rember dinner? Talking dsblity?" Vowels might flee Joe but consonants clung fast. He wanted to feel me out. He liked my work, but I hadn't ever written for theater, had I? Not really, I told him, I was just kidding around.

"Kid-ding?"

So then I thought about it. My contact with Joe and the extraordinarily influential Open Theater during the second half of its ten-year life (1963-73) had been a luminous event in my life. Their 1969 production of *The Serpent*, an interpretation of the Adam and Eve story, showed how bodies, faces, voices could trouble the line between beast and human and make palpable the opening of consciousness. Joe invited me occasionally to talk with the troupe about writing they could use in their investigations for works about dying and about mutable identity. I'd watched the troupe warm up, improvise on one another's narrated dreams, and work up material that eventually became text. (Scriptwriters here were collaborators, partly scribes.) The experience of theater as a visceral, poetic, psychophilosophical laboratory was a revelation to me.

So was the group's dynamic relation to audience, its implicit interest in the flow of social consciousness. The responses of friends at rehearsals helped shape their ever-mutable works. And when co-director Roberta Sklar brought their production of Beckett's *Endgame* to a prison where I was teaching, the audience's role was electrifying. When Clov said, "I can't be punished anymore. I'll go now to my kitchen, ten feet by ten feet by ten feet, and wait for him to whistle me," he became for this audience the prisoner—we all felt it. And, raging with contradictory authority, Hamm (played by Joe) was the warden. I'd written about the play and knew it well, but the raucous crowd's unmistakable interpretation added to its meaning.

Joe's direction of *Endgame* in Paris in 1980 prompted the reclusive Beckett to seek him out. They both wanted to empty language of meaning, and Beckett permitted Joe to adapt *Texts for Nothing* to the stage as he saw fit. After open-heart surgery caused the stroke that left Joe mute, Beckett wrote a poem for him about aphasia, *What is the word*. Their remarkable affinity seemed to me to play a role in Joe's recovery. His immersion in Beckett's elliptical language might have helped him make sense with—and perhaps bear—the eerie associative jargon with which he emerged from the stroke.

A sense of the miraculous attended Joe's recovery. In the hospital his first intelligible word was yes, even when, suicidal, he wanted to say no. Then, when it seemed that he was unlikely to regain normal speech, we realized that his theatrical bias had equipped him peculiarly well, even wordless, to continue work. An original impulse of the Open Theater, as he'd said, was to get away from talking, and the group, possessed of corporeal genius, made their bodies eloquent, while parodying speech conventions. In a sense, catastrophe crystallized what he had that he could use to survive. Joe himself appears to have recognized and taken heart from this luck buried in his misfortune.

Joe's interest in physical expressiveness, I thought, might explain his passing over some brilliant blind and deaf performers to choose for the disability workshop actors with trouble walking—those I considered, with myself, the tribe of Ahab. While fired with social, psychological ideas about our trouble, I drew a blank on our physical expressiveness. For this and other reasons, it seemed unwise to pursue this project. That sober thought made me realize how passionately I wanted to go ahead. My relation to my own body was in crisis.

Each disability story is unique, yet resonant with others. I had contracted polio through imprudence—traveling to Mexico without having taken the Salk vaccine. I was twenty-one, fresh out of college, having a last summer fling before starting graduate school—and ended up spending six months in the Sister Kenny ward at Jersey City Hospital, learning to walk all over again.

For mismatched reasons, I was not devastated. I wasn't eager to continue school just then. This affliction assuaged some of the guilt I'd felt over my older brother's mental illness. And its drama sated my super-literary imagination. Recognizing that rage and tears would be an avalanche sliding to a sea of drowning, I cultivated toughness, cool, and the absurd. Summoning the inner Bogart, I took up smoking. I invented a technique to banish feelings that ambushed me upon waking, willing them back to the far corners of the big ward. I cried only when my self-image was displaced by what I saw in the first full-length mirror.

The Sister Kenny regimen fortified this persona. I had to lie day and night on a thin mattress over a wooden bed, soles flat to the footboard, and submit to regular applications of scalding hot packs. Twice daily a man who moonlighted as a bouncer pinned down my shoulders while the physical therapist pulled my feet with such force that I expected them to tear free. It was the medieval rack, yet it made me laugh uncontrollably, instead of screaming. The absurd reflex gave me secret pleasure.

After stretching, the therapist cradled my stricken right leg, stroked where the quadriceps should contract, and instructed me to "think the motion from here." Then, repeatedly, she extended my leg with a vibrating motion. We were trying to heal the connection, severed by polio, between brain and body. Month after month, taking on all the sapped muscles, she patiently rowed my limbs. I felt only touch of finger and heartbeat of mind. One day a spark jumped, my muscle thrilled, and I saw confirmation in her eyes. This confluence of mystery and knowledge, dependency and power, stunned me. The link between our minds and wills and my body, this thinking the body, making the body think, was utopian, annealing a split older than polio. These mysteries faded, domesticated through daily drill, and my body gradually became *the* body, something *out there* to manage. Yet the rest of the treatment was powerfully formative, reinforcing my commitment to hard work, concentrated will, and optimism.

In the hospital, the release from all responsibility but to get better filled me with feverish energy—to read, write, study, sketch. The busywork of denial, this was also the mobilizing energy of survival. I never mistook it for courage. Out in the world, the reaction of others to my limp taught me a subtler form of denial. Finding a quick and casual way to say that I'd had a light case of polio, I fancied I was putting the other at ease. Of course, I was inducting him, as best I could, into the attitude I found tolerable.

My energy carried me through marriage, child-rearing, and more than thirty years of teaching, and though I limped, I ignored it and essentially forgot polio. The civil rights, anti-war, and women's movements fundamentally altered my life and work; the identity struggles of blacks, Latinos, gays, lesbians, and Native Americans stirred me. Yet I took in very little of the disability rights movement.

One day a college administrator asked me to serve on a planning committee as representative for the disabled. Why me? I wondered. I had no insight into ramps and accessible restroom stalls, as I didn't need them. So I said I didn't consider myself disabled and would not be comfortable with that task. I felt no shame, but her look said that I should. But how could I represent the disabled, I wondered defensively, and what would the slogan be? Gimpy pride?

Years later I applied for a handicapped parking permit from the city. I hated having to say, let alone prove, that I was handicapped. Once I had, a host of fresh liberties were mine. I parked at meters without paying, in front of funeral parlors and consulates, even—my wicked favorite—swell apartment buildings, despite the yellow curb and the indignation of doormen. I chauffeured friends about with panache, was the envy of alternate-side-of-the-street parking slaves. "It's disabling to own a car in New York unless you're disabled," I'd boast. I needed the permit but treated it like a scam. From cringing inhibition, I'd advanced to gimpy arrogance—though not to pride.

I was riding on a movement for which I hadn't lifted a finger.

Then in the 1990s I discovered weakness in my left leg, until then apparently sound, though it had been paralyzed for three days at first. I had trouble with stairs and often, for no reason, was assailed by fatigue. I learned that this was post-polio syndrome, in which the old polio-vanquishing formula, "use it or lose it," was reversed; now excessive exercise could cause permanent muscle loss.

More than the changing of habits, a transformation of personality and ethos was demanded. People counseled me to "listen to my body," little knowing how unacquainted with its idiom I was. I had coped by transcendence—escaping, denying, or subordinating the limits of the flesh—and this was now impossible. My body was in full mutiny, shouting, but I couldn't catch the message. Maybe, I thought, just maybe, if I could abandon my reliance on determination, or change its direction, give up the notion of intellectual "mastery" (a notion which feminism had critiqued, but not eliminated from my mind-body regime), I would move past the triumphalism which had divided me from my own flesh as well as from others with bodies in trouble.

Never had I so needed people who had come to terms with disability. Yet I was uneasy around strangers who seemed "worse off" than me, for half-consciously I'd built my confidence on such distinctions. I'd cultivated a physical snobbery which I'd have to overcome if I was to learn to attend to my own body. Yet I was scared to admit that my edge was eroding. Now I knew what it was to have guts, and I fell short.

Thinking this way made working with Joe more alluring. Beyond his remarkable adaptation, there was the privileging the body over thought—or refusal of the separation—that distinguished his work. And Joe's heart disease had made death his familiar. The Open Theater's *Terminal* had mocked the American cult of evasion of mortal reality. His preference for process over product, for liminal states and fluid identities—all reflected a sense of transience. Sometimes his work served to push back the dark, or allowed us to enter it and believe we might survive. Along with functional loss, the symbolic weight of disability, its intimation of death, is what makes us fear and loathe it. With Joe, we might begin to accept and integrate our mortality.

So I said, Yes, if Joe would take a chance with me, I'd grab it. With no long-term goals in theater, I had little to lose, even if I fell on my face as a writer. I had ideas I wanted to explore, and my resistance to facing disability might help me engage and shake up the audience's resistance. But I had no illusions about my primary motive. I was in it for myself; I felt compelled. Joe might understand that—wasn't that how he worked?

Anders Cato, Joe's assistant, and the dramaturg Bill Hart, both active in the project from the beginning, were practiced in fathoming Joe's wishes from ambiguous clues. The three of them filled me in. Joe had found their 1992 work too light; that of 1993 too heavy. Asked what he wanted, Joe enunciated, "Fun-ny." "Like cabaret?" I asked, and he brightened. "Or vaudeville?" someone ventured, and he was gleeful. "Yes! Fun-ny." But not trivial. Nor sentimental or politically correct—that went without saying. An upbeat play about handicaps won Joe's withering verdict: "High-school." He had weaned himself from despair by contemplating stars; he'd draw out the word in awe—*stars*. Vastness still drew him. "'Fun-ny' and 'stars'", Bill summarized. "It's Joe's haiku." All three seemed stymied, yet hopeful that a fresh theatrical attack or a unifying theme—something magical or probing—might make the project go.

Magical, probing—that sounded right for my own double riddle: how to heed / accept / care for my weakening body, how to move honestly toward the damaged flesh of others. Magic might be the probe; probing might provide magical entry into a new perspective. I read Oliver Sacks, the magician who probes neurological aberrations and revolutionizes our sense of them. Rejecting the category "illness," Sacks shows that, if we suspend our faith in norms, we find in persons with "physical deficits" a wealth of adaptive strengths, novel powers, sometimes an organic culture with its own idiom. The creation by the deaf of Sign, a vibrant language with qualities lacking in our noisy tongue, was simply the most literal example. In *A Leg to Stand On*, Sacks uncovered no such culture, for his own leg injury was unique. Our tribe of Ahab had divergent medical histories. Might we yet have a common culture?

Talking with the actors, I pursued such questions. Ray Robertson was a twenty-year-old Marine outside Khe Sanh when he tripped the booby trap that took one leg off below the knee. The narrative style of this tall, rangy, fair-haired man reflects his droll spirit. "I was on patrol, walking point, when suddenly I was airborne. There's a thump and I was laying there, and I heard a blood-curdling scream. I said to myself, Holy Shit, is that you? I didn't have the answer, but I knew whoever was screaming was hurting, and I was hoping it wasn't me." People had been dying all around him, and when he was flying home, he said, "I'm like, the war is over, baby! Nothing in the *world* can bring me down. It's not a million-dollar wound, but it's good enough. I'm not going to get killed."

This buoyant, generous response to trouble is Ray's signature. Back in Plattsburgh, New York, with a prosthetic foot, he bought a motorcycle, then a Corvette, "anything that went fast. I didn't think I was going to live to be twenty-one. I didn't care. I didn't have any respect or fear, what were they going to do to me? Did I want to die? Nah, I just didn't care." He liked living on the edge. "When I came home, I took flying lessons," Ray said. And went gliding. "They tow me in the air, let the bird fly free. You hit a thermal and go up, up, up. Then *straight* down, the ground coming at you. Whew!"

Knowing something of that ebullient physical recklessness, I told Ray how flying haunted me after polio. And Robert F. Murphy dedicated *The Body Silent*, about his experience of quadriplegia, "to all those who cannot walk—and instead try to fly." Arnold Beisser, the tennis champion thrust by polio into an iron lung, called his memoir *Flying Without Wings*. Could it be that our bodies, disqualified from being ordinary, could only be extraordinary? I told Ray that Sacks, lacking an inner image of his injured leg, felt that he had forgotten his personal "motor" music until listening to a recording of Mendelssohn one day, his "kinetic melody" returned, "somehow elicited by, and attuned to, the Mendelssohnian melody." Though Sacks's condition was particular, I wondered whether all of us hadn't had to rediscover, or reinvent, a kinetic melody. Ray told me that, after getting his prosthetic, "I didn't want to appear abnormal, so I made the good limb match the other." As if hearkening to the kinetic melody in the new foot, the old came to harmonize. His bracemaker calls him a "master of compensation" because he adapts to each new foot. Though his father urged him to get a desk job, Ray had no sooner arrived in New York and seen *Sleuth* than he fixed on acting. He studied at the Neighborhood Playhouse School of Theater and acted with the Veterans Ensemble Theater Company off-Broadway. But "Vetco got bogged down in war—it was the downfall of the company." Living with his wife Jayne, a pediatrician, and four kids on Staten Island, Ray minimizes his disability. He avoids reserved parking-spots: "I leave them for someone who's really disabled."

Although she qualifies as "really disabled," Anita Hollander creates the opposite impression. She was immersed in theater when disaster struck. Born to the stage—one grandmother in vaudeville, another in the Cleveland Orchestra, her father a cantor—she has performed professionally since she was eight. She was studying acting at Carnegie-Mellon when cancer was detected in her leg. When the tumor was removed, she traumatically lost her voice. Assisting Kristin Linklater, a teacher who'd written about voice and the body, Anita said, "I learned from the inside out what voice is about, I got a bodied awareness of voice." She recovered a deeper voice with a range, husky to crystalline, that suits her emotional reach, from poignancy to chutzpah. "I'm the least fragile person in the world," she said. A huge grin widened her heart-shaped face.

In 1982, after studying in Europe, Anita was in Boston, at twenty-six directing and rehearsing in *Jacques Brel is Alive and Well and Living in Paris.* The cancer recurred, bringing excruciating pain. When she guessed that her leg would have to be amputated, she begged her doctor to do it quickly, so the show could open on schedule four weeks after the operation. "Everyone thought I was crazy, but I said, 'They're amputating my leg, not my brain!'" Besides, "I was dragging around a dead limb, I was ready to say good-bye and get on with life." Show biz discipline saw her through. "I was ready to perform every night, because that was my survival, to have that goal. I knew that after the eight-week run I could fall apart. And I did. I regressed, I took myself back through the whole experience. She laughed. "I have a tendency to monitor my experience—'that's really interesting! I think I'll take notes!'"

While teaching at NYU, Anita took two writing workshops, taking heavy criticism for work based on her ordeal. "But getting hammered by other writers helped me move away and develop on my own." Working at the Comedy Club seated on the piano without her prosthesis gave her confidence. "The improv audience is the hardest crowd there is. If you can turn them toward you, you can do anything." There she wrote her punning song about hating physical therapy until she got a walkman ("I can move, move, move / I'm getting in the groove / of a walkman!

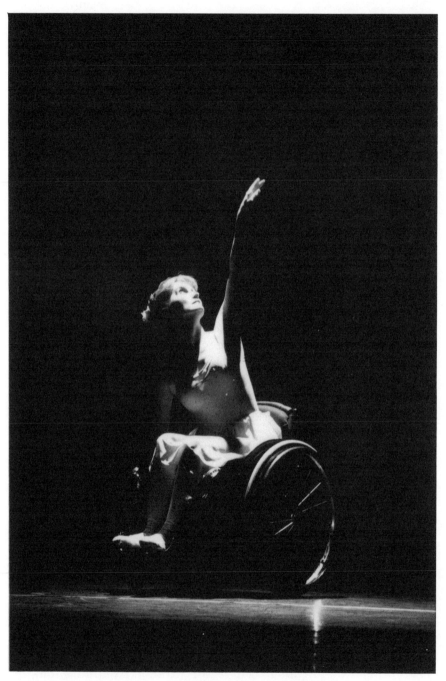

KITTY LUNN
Photo: James Estrin for the *New York Times*

. . . I got no time to talk / I gotta walk, man") for her cabaret show, *Still Standing.*

Anita married actor Paul Hamilton ("he thought it was cool that I had one leg") and bore a daughter, Holland. When a three-year-old, observing Anita's one-legged swimming, concluded she was a mermaid, Anita wrote a song, "Mommy is a Mermaid," for Holland. "Nourished in countless ways" by Holland, Anita takes her everywhere she can. Such support helps explain her radiant, large-spirited stage presence. The in-your-face humor is her own. Songs like "Why I prefer one" (on having to shave only one leg, find only one sock), suggest a survival strategy: she will jar us into seeing her on her own terms—or swiftly do without us. The 1992 workshop inspired that song and one with the rousing chorus, "Hey! That's the way it is! but cripples ain't supposed to be happy!" (I too favor for myself the blunt accuracy of this unfashionable term—as does the writer Nancy Mairs.)

Like Anita, Kitty Lunn has reshaped her career around disability. If her mother had had her way, she'd have raised her diminutive fine-featured daughter with flaming hair as a New Orleans belle. But Kitty's widowed grandmother could repair roofs and cars and taught her that she could do whatever she set her mind to. Seeing *The Red Shoes* at eight inspired Kitty to dance her way out of a difficult household. She won a scholarship to the Washington School of Ballet, soloed in the National Ballet, and became an actress. About to perform on Broadway in 1987, she fell down a flight of icy steps and broke her back. After five operations, she learned she would never walk again. "I thought my life was over. But my grandmother always said, 'Life is going to go on with you or without you—so you'd better get on with it.'" Ironically, she says, "Not being able to work was not the hardest part, but rather to keep hold of my identity as a sexually-functioning woman. I had to fight for that." She married actor Andrew Macmillan and became an activist. "Andrew says my legacy will be the Kitty Lunn memorial toilets I got installed throughout the theater district."

Improvising for the 1992 disability workshop, Kitty showed how Luigi, a disabled dancer, had taught her to work from the rhythm of the body. As she was demonstrating in her chair, she asked Anita to sing and kept moving. "It was an extraordinary moment. I knew I had to keep dancing. I had never before imagined I could dance in a chair." Later she joined the Cleveland

Dancing Wheels. When I mentioned Sacks's "kinetic melody," Kitty said, "There's a dancer inside me who doesn't know or care that I broke my back. She keeps dancing and waiting for me to catch up. Being a dancer has as much to do with what you have inside as what your legs can do."

Adversity made Anita and Kitty, like Joe and Ray, sharpen and deepen a core of their identity. Singing, acting, dancing since childhood, these women's bodies had been their expressive instruments, and so they remained when each transvalued the damage done her. On one leg, Anita enlarges her bold, full-bodied, vitality; while Kitty fashions grace in novel terms. Because polio had made me turn from the physical to the political and literary, their different self-transformations thrilled me and lifted a depression I hadn't quite realized was there.

Unlike the others, Jan Kissick was born with disability, the cerebral palsy that slightly impairs his gait. Jan's curly hair and tender features made him look younger than his thirty years, and his intense confiding manner underscored his vulnerable air. His first words in the workshop, delivered with a hoarse rural-Oklahoma twang—"I'd be an asshole without c.p."—made me invite him for a drink to hear more. As an adolescent in the little town of Cache (named for the legend that the James brothers hid their loot in its mountains), he told me, "I was tortured. Other kids stuck me in a trash can, threw bottles of piss on my head." He lost himself in movies—"I could quote huge chunks of a movie after seeing it once"—but did not consider acting. In his world, "arts were for fags," and Jan felt his looks were a liability. Then he saw John Malkovich in a TV presentation of *True West*. "His talent was electrifying, and he was not pretty." At the American Academy of Dramatic Arts in New York, as Jan describes it, the training was naturalistic and stressed the actors' relation to each other. Bartending at the Plymouth Theater when Lanford Wilson's *Burn This!* was on, Malkovich's performance again moved Jan. "He opened me up to the need for theatricality, for connecting with the audience." With this revised sense of acting, Jan's disability came to seem a boon. "It helps me keep my feet on the ground. Without it, I'd be too full of myself or could lose myself in art. I don't want to stand above others. I'd be less able to translate. . . . I don't want to masturbate on the stage, I want to have sex." Putting it another way, he said, "I want to work for the kid in the audience who's missing something."

Jan told the group about meeting a terrific woman at a bar, really hitting it off. After some drinks, Jan had to go to the bathroom, but the woman would see his feet! He plotted a course between tables to conceal his gait, but there was no avoiding his first exposing steps. He excused himself, didn't look back, and wondered if she would still be there when he returned. (She was, as it happened.) Jan's relative ability to "pass" for "normal" set him apart from the other actors, and complicated his self-identification as disabled. His unresolved social anguish prompts his best work. My similar turmoil—I didn't yet fully "belong" to the disabled class—drew me to Jan.

Two nondisabled actors joined the project in 1992, partly to act as surrogates for the audience, partly to avoid "quarantining" the disabled. Charlotte Colavins is witty, dark and small, and Wayne Maugans, blond and strapping. Their unusual gifts of empathy and improvisation enriched their contributions to the group's exploration. A darkly comic imagination emerged in Wayne's improvisations on disturbed fantasies of the nondisabled and Charlotte's on the madness near the surface of both fit and disabled.

Shortly before the 1994 workshop began, Public Theater people introduced Joe to Barry Martin. The injustice inherent in tales of calamity attains mythic proportions in Barry's story. Raised in the Bronx in a West Indian family, Barry had just graduated from SUNY-Purchase in 1983 and was dancing with a British troupe in Sun City, a homeland set up as an entertainment resort exempt from South Africa's apartheid laws. On a day off, Barry accompanied a white dancer to a dentist and had an automobile accident. An ambulance picked up the white man, leaving Barry behind. Black passersby took him to the emergency room of a whites-only hospital, but he was not served. Sun City officials arranged his transfer to a hospital for blacks in Pretoria. Riding seventy-five miles of bumpy road without having his neck secured, Barry was quadriplegic upon arrival. Because the black hospital lacked necessary facilities, he was given, as an American, "honorary white" status and transferred to another hospital.

After a year's hospitalization in England, Barry got an M.A. at N.Y.U. He started a dance company, heartbreakingly called Déjà Vu, while transforming himself into a choreographer. The Brooklyn Academy of Music, City Center, the Joyce Theater and

Lincoln Center have featured his work, and Alvin Ailey commissioned a dance piece. Barry was (and is) working on an autobiographical musical with George Wolfe. Seeing him in his motorized chair, tall, graceful, austerely handsome in dreadlocks, one could forget his loss and, say, pass him a sheet of paper—until his low "put it in my lap!" startled one to awareness. Joe told me that the notion of a disability theater piece initially put Barry off. How this formidably reserved young man would collaborate was not clear when we gathered at the Public Theater.

Yet it was Barry who got us started that first day.

In his telegraphic way, Joe said we'd use our first week for improvisation, the second for pulling together a public presentation. He intimated how open the project still was, saying it might be called The Cripple-God, or the Island, or Eclipse, or something else. He asked me to talk about my ideas. Eclipse sounds good, I said. I'd been thinking that, since all of us but Jan had been violently changed as adults, a narrative frame might be a U-shaped journey, a passage from the light down to dark and back up to the light. We'd move from a position of unconscious privilege, or health, through radical disorientation and isolation, then through a series of comic and shocking misunderstandings with the nondisabled, to complete alienation. At the nadir, we'd begin to discover each other and the culture of our tribe, the tribe of Ahab. Though loathing our broken selves and fellow outcasts, through some ritual of initiation we'd work our way to mutual affirmation, self-acceptance, and ascent. We'd draw on rituals of reversal, of excess and exception—like Carnival, with its wild transgressions, its overturned hierarchies, the beggar becoming king, the grotesque, beautiful. Or like the Bacchanal, the drunken orgy where you transcend ordinary consciousness and lose distinctions of identity, gender—even species. In Euripides' play, the Bacchantes rent bodies limb from limb in ecstasy. I wondered, did Ray or Anita have extra prostheses?

"That's like the underworld journey the shaman has to take to become a healer," Gabrielle Roth, a movement consultant, put in. Having invented her own kind of dancing after injuring her knee, Gabrielle is a kind of shamanic Bacchante herself; she leads workshops where participants dance out their inner lives.

Then, describing Sacks's kinetic melody idea and Ray's adaptation to his prosthetic, I suggested that awkwardness might be

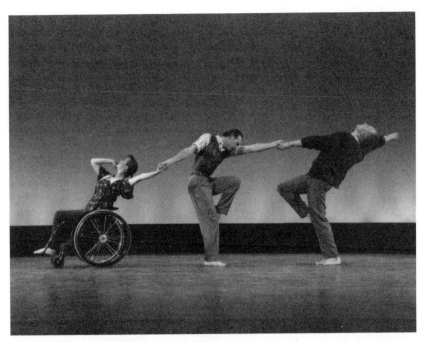

"Dancing Out Their Inner Lives." Scene from a performance of the Infinity Dance Theater featuring Kitty Lunn, Robert Koval, and Christopher Nelson.

transformed into a personal dance. Joe picked it up and called for the first exercise: "Awkward to graceful." Gabrielle put on a New Age tape, full of drums, flutes, and birdcalls. Everyone began to contrive rhythms around rigid limbs or tics, Wayne and Charlotte rotated around invented deformities. In their chairs Kitty careened and Barry made tiny moves. The effect was atomized, strange, rather more awkward than graceful.

Then Barry suggested they enter the performance space one at a time, connect somehow with the people already there, create a picture. This time they formed tentative couples and triangles, dissolved and regrouped, gradually settling into a tableau. With his unreadable impassivity—was he indifferent? superior? or simply serene?—Barry stretched out his arms at his sides and remained still. He looked as though he had sublimated all pain, and as the dancers were drawn to him, he commanded a small constellation. Jan crouched and knelt at the side of his chair, abjectly embraced and kissed the wheel, then threw back his head in a silent howl under Barry's sheltering arm. Everyone froze.

The rest of us were stunned, glimpsing the project's mysterious potential.

The potential was never realized. The workshop advanced chaotically. Anita was performing elsewhere the first two days, Kitty the second week. Joe or Bill, the dramaturg, would assign homework but not always find time to look at it. An aphasic painter or a philosopher with cerebral palsy might address us instead; or Bill might abruptly shift gears in hopes of jarring the actors into something "bold" or "dangerous." We seemed at cross-purposes, Bill after the sexy or perverse, Joe the eccentric or poetic (but not heavy), I the light through the darkness.

One night over dinner I poured out to Joe how much Open Theater explorations of painful, fearful experience had meant to me. "You made it possible, safe, for the audience to look at things we hadn't imagined we could dare—or bear—to see." He heard me out, then shrugged. "I'm changed. Fun-ny now." He ducked his head with a throaty conspiratorial laugh, nudging me so I shouldn't take it hard. I was disappointed, especially because his old work was what had drawn me there. But I still puzzle over this difference. Was I, who had comparatively only sipped despair, naive about how much pain I could handle? Could Joe, having drunk deep of suicidal depression, have willfully simplified his feelings in order to go on? Or had he reached a different profundity? His brooding restlessness had apparently yielded to a sweet acceptance. Why should I doubt the depth of his capacity for humor, even joy?

Our debate was moot. On the third day, Joe told us that interested Public Theater people could attend a presentation only on Thursday, eight days later. "Too everything fast now," he complained. It was immensely frustrating. Rather than develop some of the promising new things, like the first day's tableau, the actors had to recreate half-forgotten bits from 1992 and polish a handful of new pieces. My eclipse narrative did not govern the final offering, but our investigations shed light on every stage of my proposed journey. Here, rescued from my notebooks, our conversations, the presentation, and our cutting-room floor, is how.

The change: the fall from grace

How to dramatize the passage from blissful, ignorant, bodily health, to incomprehensible loss or alteration? How stage the mind's shock at finding itself slave to the body, or emotional alienation so great that one can't recognize one's scream or translate it into laughter?

Joe's exercise: wake up and find your body changed. Wayne, on trying to dress, found his clothes grotesquely shrunken. Ray woke up with his foot become a flipper. Wayne's most brilliant conceit was discovering his limbs moved only backwards. Slowly getting the hang of it, he holds his trousers behind him, and jumps backwards into his shoes. He played it deadpan, absorbed by detail, oblivious to implications.

How enact the soul's desire to refuse the unacceptable flesh? I sketched a routine: *A wheelchaired mime tries to abandon her body, become pure spirit. She hypnotizes herself with a mantra. But the body keeps interrupting, pulls her down. She pauses and reflects. She tries to fool gravity, with one spring from the waist up, leave the body behind. Failure. She pauses and reflects. She seeks to escape species-identity, replace earth as a medium. When flapping arms fail to gain the air, she tries side-stroke, back stroke, breast-stroke, and crawl. She pauses and reflects. She begins a striptease, slowly discards her clothes, then continues with the flesh, trying to unzip torso, untie feet, unbutton the cuffs of wrists, unscrew hands, work fingers off one by one, as with a glove; growing frantic, she tries to peel off scalp like bathing-cap, unbuckle legs. Broken into fragments, this scene could be repeated intermittently. The mime finally inflicts murderous rage on her treacherous body, then, in horrific recoil, begs forgiveness, cradles her flesh, croons over it.*

Anita approached reconciliation with her amputated leg differently in her song, "Funeral for a Replaceable Part." "Even sick you carried me / Through Europe's ice and snow. You let me keep dancing / Now how can I let you go? . . . Sorry for the pain / Hope it's better where you are."

How to come to love one's body's strangeness? Jan told a story, beginning typically in left field. "My girlfriend and I were rarely alone in my parents' house. But once we had sex on the stairs, and I saw her looking at my feet. I'm self-conscious about my feet. But when I was studying in New York, I lived at the Y and used to run around the track a lot, sometimes at three in the morning. I ran toe-to-heel because of the c.p. After about a year my toenails turned black and fell off. Before, I considered my feet my enemy (I was in my head), but when my nails grew back three times as thick, I thought, evolution usually takes thousands of years, this happened in two. Now I see my feet as good guys working to help the whole me."

The world's intervention: becoming its thing

We rarely get time and privacy to adapt to loss and naturalize in our newly alien flesh. The damaged body belongs first to everyone else. At every stage, the big-eyed others interrupt one's solitary adaptation and make transcendence impossible. We encounter our change in their eyes, but with urgencies different from our own.

First doctors. All of us knew the devastating objectification of doctors on "grand rounds." My doctor would sweep in, tails of his white coat flying, with an entourage of visitors, would hold forth and sweep away again. I was not introduced. If I tried to tell of my progress in physical therapy, the doctor's condescension was withering. (The writer Ynestra King told me that when the doctors descended, she'd pipe up, "Let me do it. This seven-year-old female has poliomyelitis, with paralysis from the gluteus maximus to the lower extremities. . . .") My swallowed rancor bore fruit in a series of "dances with doctors" that I wrote up for Joe. (*The patient answers the doctor's questions but the doctor tells the attendants, "You see, her mind's affected, she can't make any sense. Hopeless." Again, she tries to get his attention in English, then Italian, then Chinese; he hears nothing. Again, raging, she addresses him as he did her, as if he were a thing. And so on.*) Fun-ny? Joe's veto was swift. "Hosptl, doctor, no, depressing."

So be it. The mere writing of these scenes, retrieving the body's memory, was cathartic. Besides, the non-medical world's responses provide ample absurd material. In them, these innocents betray their superstitions. Some touch us cripples for good luck (their own, of course, not ours). Others cross themselves or count their rosaries at the sight of us. In the workshop, Kitty cited the Greeks—cripples make better lovers—but noted that media stereotypes are malevolent. "Hunchbacks are assumed to be vengeful, like Dr. Strangelove. Women are passive or manipulative, or both." Jan thought it just as oppressive to cast cripples as superheroes or saints. "They think you're nice because you're in a chair. No one wants to pay to see a piece called 'Crippled Boy has shitty day'." Someone quoted Linda Hunt in *The Year of Living Dangerously*: "Being a dwarf means you can be smarter than anyone else and no one will envy you." Kitty concurred. "In a chair I can get away with murder." Jan: "Yeah, how come there's not a show called 'Disabled serial killer'?"

We talked of the invasiveness and appropriativeness of strangers. They seem to assume we've no right to privacy or will be grateful for any attention. Trespass betrays their anxiety. When Joe asked a visiting aphasic stroke victim what was the stupidest thing people do, she said simply, "LOUD!" This stimulated the gratifying assignment to collect "stupid questions." Nothing brought us into such raucous rapport as this collective retaliation. The result was the "Questions" routine which opens this essay. There were more:

> *"Is there a telethon for that?"*
> *"If you swim with one leg, do you go in circles?"*
> *"Have you heard of the power of Nam Yoho Renge Kyo?"*
> *"You know, you can reverse Karma."*
> *"So . . . where is your leg, actually?"*
> *"I know what you're going through."*

We had more material than we could use. When Jan was out with his girlfriend, someone asked, "What happened to *her*?" Barry said, "It pisses me off when people act like I'm invisible." Kitty recalled the marriage clerk's admonishment, "I hope you appreciate that he's marrying you anyhow!" and the psychiatrist's remark, "I assume your husband is homosexual." We are the occasion of primitive fantasies and phobias which, at their worst, coincide in cruel prurience. Someone's favorite outrageous question, "Is there anything you would like to ask me about life?", for all its smug gentility, is on a continuum with the shifty-eyed whisper, "Can you have orgasms?" Barry told us how a stranger, an elderly white woman, helped him and his friends find a table in a crowded restaurant and sent them champagne. Later she came to ask, "May I kiss you?" "Before I could answer, she had darted her tongue into my mouth."

Barry's story reminded me of a 1992 workshop exercise I'd heard about. Joe's task was to improvise something with another actor without telling the other in advance; meanwhile Bill had been saying, "Let's go darker." "I brought in a tape of musical bits I'd strung together," Wayne told me. "It began with flowery music. I went up to Kitty with a basket of rose-petals, sprinkled them over her, and acted flirtatious. The music turned ominous. I took some rope and tied her hands to the wheelchair. Then, with a plastic stage switchblade, I stroked under her chin. I circled one of her breasts. The music changed again, I got on my knees. She was in bare feet, and I started smelling, kissing, sucking her foot. The music then became an alleluia chorus, a glorious angelic thing. I started crying and ended up trying to redeem myself and released her."

Completely unprepared, Kitty was very upset, and the improvisation was dropped. But many people told me how powerfully disturbing it was. (To Wayne as well: though he'd kept it to himself in 1992, he confided recently that he'd been working through an early experience of sexual abuse. "It had been disabling to me mentally and emotionally; that was really why I was there.") In his daring, Wayne had revealed how the presence of damaged, powerless flesh can destabilize the nondisabled and pose an erotic temptation. His performance suggested that disability calls up the carnal (the underside of chivalric romance) in the viewer, and simultaneously a conviction of relative power that can become sadistic. The combined vulnerability and strangeness of the disabled triggers a feeling of exception and license in the other and obliterates awareness of the disabled person's interiority. (When the powerless one is black or female, the dynamic is reinforced.)

Reinventing social selves: defense, revenge, and shadowing

Society makes us all take roles. But we fallen ones are under particularly intense pressure to assuage the world's manifold anxiety—or fend it off. Disaster forces us on stage. I'd begun my cripple career as a cheerful pedagogue, volunteering the information to the curious. But I wearied of this role. Sometimes a stranger's thoughtless "What happened to your leg?" shattered my distraction, reminded me of my forgotten aberration, and tempted me to reply, "And what misfortunes have you had?" (A workshop colleague proposed the malicious retort, "What happened to your face?")

Gentle Kitty has been pressed to perform her outrage. When, say, waiting in line at a bus-stop in her chair, a man approaches and whispers, "Do you mind if I ask—Can you still have sex?" she has learned to turn to the crowd around and ask at the top of her lungs, "Can you believe what this person just asked me?"

Retaliation offers short-lived relief; if we give no better than we get, we fail to alter the terms of encounter. I wondered: If we weren't forced out of ourselves to appease the public terror or to defend or revenge ourselves on its intrusion, could we change the nature of our exchange? (All of us are blessed with friends and family who see us more nearly as we are; at issue here are the anonymous Able Bodies.) If we could set the terms, what might they be? Does our fall from grace, like the Biblical Fall, bring special knowledge? Does it give us an edge?

Our history is written on our bodies, but Able Bodies appear to be blank slates. Health and wholeness are wasted on Able Bodies, as youth is on the young. The ABs, as I began to fancy them, are ignorant of all but the first letters of the body's alphabet. Not having to know the body, to think every motion, they seem, ironically, less evolved. Moreover, through the lens of our special consciousness, we see their fear of mortality and terror of dependency, heightened in a culture that equates loss of self-reliance with death. We are an unenviable vanguard, but a vanguard nonetheless. Can our changed state—once we have accepted it— give us superior appreciation of vulnerability and interdependence? Can we re-vision our relationship with the others? Are we deficient—or they, because we know the body's secret destiny that they shrink from? Are we their spooks, their haunting fears? Or, like the leg the amputee cannot believe is gone and calls a phantom, are their intact bodies our phantoms? How to break through the mutually crippling hierarchy, how convey that we are each other's shadows, one flesh?

In a subtle pas de deux, Wayne and Anita played the ancient mirror game. "It's almost a cliché, an exercise for Acting 101," Wayne told me. Facing each other, they tipped heads simultaneously toward the audience, then away, raised mirroring arms, waved and circled them, thrust them on matching hips, and so on. Then they both made a twisting gesture at the hip joint, but Anita unhooked her artificial leg and let it fall to the floor. Peo-

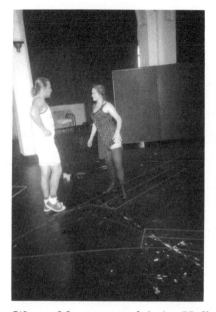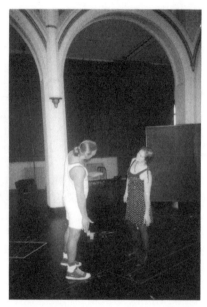

Wayne Maugans and Anita Hollander playing the ancient mirror game. Photos by Bell Gale Chevigny.

ple watching gasped, then laughed uncomfortably. For a boggling moment Wayne seemed incapacitated, limited in human expressiveness. Not to be outdone, he lifted one leg and stood on the other. But when he lost his balance, he went off in a huff, while she remained standing, hopping gracefully for balance, beaming. (Later, while Jan drummed, Anita danced like a wild dervish on her solo leg, further de-stabilizing the viewers.)

In "Double," Jan and Wayne played with misconceptions (and real bonds) between the apparently "normal" and the other. Jan sparked the idea when he told me how much he liked Wayne, who shares his taste in women and music and had survived by tending the same bars. Wayne concurred: "We're the same age, have similar backgrounds, both grew up in the country, Jan is a real buddy." "If I could make myself over," Jan said with his disarming candor, "I'd be Wayne. He's my alter-ego." One day we three got together to explore this affinity. Wayne recalled a famous improv exercise Viola Spolin had designed called "giving voice," where Actor 1, say, stands behind actor 2, and whispers words that Actor 2 delivers almost simultaneously. Actor 2,

Wayne explained, "doesn't have to think about the lines but acts them, with a feeling of surprise." One body concealing another who sparks the speech of the first struck me as an uncanny expression of linkage, alter-egohood, and the arbitrariness of identity. I suggested that each stand behind the other to whisper what he imagined the other felt.

"What I want most in the whole world," Wayne whispered, and Jan spoke, "is to be like you, to wake up in the morning and look in the mirror and see myself and be proud of who I am, to have my legs be straight, to have my body be slender and strong and virile, to have women desire me."

Then Jan whispered, Wayne said, "You have no idea how—*fine*—it feels to walk down the street every day knowing that every head turns when I walk past, hearing that little [gasp] catch of breath, knowing that no matter what the light is like, my cheekbones are making the most of it." Delivering the halting phrases, Wayne seemed astonished and enchanted by narcissism. "My looks are something I carry with me like a *prize*—I love them so much! I know you'd all like to be me, every single one of you, man, woman, and child, disabled and able-bodied. Wouldn't you like to come up, one by one, and touch my hair?"

Now say what you really feel about yourself, I suggested. Wayne whispered his confession, and Jan delivered it. "It's really not all that. When I wake up I don't feel rested. I look in the mirror, I look like a piece of shit, you smoked too much last night, you're getting fat, you haven't worked out enough, your back is killing me, you just are not what you used to be, God! I'd love to be taller, to have dark hair, strong virile muscles. I wish I was witty, I wish I was aggressive, I wish I weren't so—ummnn—nice!"

They changed places and Jan whispered. "The way you see me, it's not me, not the real me. You see the shambling, the stumbling, the lunge, and you don't see me. I'd like to be you, have women desire me. Except for the feet, I'm almost you. But most of all, I'd like a chance, just one chance to show you the way I see myself, the way I know I am. It's not that bad once you get used to it. Please, just a day, no, not that—a minute, a second, a *second*—that's all I need, a *second*—you would all love me."

We were thrilled. The deflected speech gave them permission to hear and confess multiple fantasy. The piece gave form to the fluid, mingling dance of longing and social perception. They repeated it later for the group. Joe called it perfect, and—playing out his idea of eclipse, I thought—showed them how to rotate around each other between speeches. Bill liked only the first half, and wanted "Wayne's" vanity to have the last word—"I'm still better!" I argued we'd lose all the richness that way, but Bill said the second half didn't "play." I thought Bill was too dependent on getting a laugh, afraid to risk a plea for sympathy, confusing it with sentimentality; he thought I lacked a theatrical sense. In the end, they did only half but without Wayne's reductive retort.

Engaging ourselves together

Solitary efforts to re-inhabit our altered bodies and relocate ourselves in the world through protective personae or strengthened bonds to the nondisabled carry us only so far. My hunch from the start was that we could more deeply accept our altered bodies and the changed world by embracing each other in our strangeness. Watching and talking with the actors confirmed it many times over.

First was the chance to work with Joe. His reputation, even after the stroke, attracted all the actors. "He has such a brilliant mind, and nothing holds him back," Wayne said. "He encouraged me to take risks and gave me permission to fail." Joe's provocative question, "who do you hate?", spurred Wayne to address his disabling abuse experience. And the other actors showed him the value in overcoming obstacles.

Barry said, "acting was the furthest thing from my mind" when he met Joe, but he was drawn by what he knew of him and of the Open Theater philosophy, "going down different roads rather than down this avenue." Accustomed, post-accident, to a back-stage role, Barry wasn't ready, he said, "to go in front of the scenes. A lot of that had to do with ego and with how society defines who should be hidden away in closets." In the workshop's final meeting, he told us he'd been "wowed by all the talent in the room," and daunted because he was no actor. But, for an exercise on narrating accidents, Barry adapted West-Indian and African-American accents to punchy and sinister street monologues—on a treacherous dope-dealer, for instance, or a gangster whose code bars squealing. "The monologues had nothing to do with me, and I got away from role models, too. I liked being able to deal with real issues in an atmosphere of magic. We were going all the way out there. It was a pain and a pleasure to

see through people and the way they react to someone disabled."
The experience "opened up possibilities that I didn't know existed and brought my artistry to another level."

"Barry wasn't even an actor," Anita exclaimed, "but he did such strong characters!" So she created a nihilist whose response to loss was the opposite of hers, "except of course everyone we create is a part of us." Barry also inspired Charlotte to dare portraying someone disabled. Her monologue as an aphasic—drawing on intimate memories of her father's stroke—was one of the most moving in the presentation.

Anita spoke glowingly of Ray. She'd learned in her one-woman show "how to grab an audience through comedy, but Ray's intelligence, intensity, and talent, she said, "invited the audience in from all angles." Though his experience of amputation was different, his understanding helped her dramatize her phantom pain. Their rapport led to an audacious collaboration. "Ray and I had the same idea," Anita explained. "It was just a question of who was going to say it first." In the skit, Ray and Anita fall into a steamy embrace, then onto a mattress. From under the covers, they toss out their clothes, shoes, underclothes, then his prosthetic, then hers, finally a third. "We generated a fifth leg," Anita says. Though the piece was scrapped, it emboldened me to pursue my idea of interchangeable or merging limbs.

My chance came the day Joe passed me a note: "Anita is glad to music for words. She's ready." Yes, he said, he wanted me to write a song. For tomorrow. Yes, it could be on what we called my Carnival of the Gimps. But for tomorrow! The U-shaped journey, when I'd described it the first day, had been a solution, intuitive but theoretical, to the problem of advancing from self-hating isolation to connection with others and self-affirmation. But being with the group made me feel its rightness. I'd heard it in Ray's exclamation, "There's no way disability can keep talented people down!" and in Kitty's assertion that if someone found a cure for her spine, she'd hesitate. I'd felt it in Barry's palpable warming to the group, in Jan's canny creeping to Barry's wheel to howl beneath his extended arm, in Jan and Wayne's affinity, in Wayne's dangerous daring with Kitty, in Ray's and Anita's erotic tossing of limbs. I'd watched Kitty make a bus kneel to scoop up her wheelchair and Anita speed down the street one-legged on her crutches at top-speed, saying gaily, "I'm much more comfortable this way than on my prosthetic!" I'd been touched by Jan's confessed affection for his evolutionary toenails. And their physical self-acceptance was comforting and contagious. Around them, I'd felt a visceral freedom to move in an easier, less decorous way and to fling my limbs around to Gabrielle's wild music in our warm-ups. Some inner guard came down, and, with the release, a taste of exhilarating peacefulness. *We have these bodies* —it occurred to me in the middle of the night—*this life, in common.* I was ready, too.

At home that night, I took down *The Bacchae* to re-read, but went instead to ask a neighbor and her visitor from Rio about their enthusiasm for Brazilian Carnival. They described fabulous reversals and glorious license—people dancing in clothes so large you can't tell if they're male or female, and fat women in bikinis. They talked about seeing through others' eyes and dancing on others' feet, being consumed by the moment and losing all sense of time, mixing with the multitude and shaking off individual identity, feeling eros more powerfully than sex. "You are freed by the flesh from the flesh," one pronounced. Back in my apartment. I poured myself a glass of wine to invoke Bacchus' help, wrote a few lines, and promptly fell asleep.

When I woke at four a.m., the song was waiting, nudged into life by dream-fragments of Lear, Andrew Marvell, shamanism, and even the Aztec sacrifice. To my surprise, Joe liked it, everyone did. Joe passed the words to Anita, with the adjuration, "Not too sentimental." I said I imagined music close to speech throughout but advancing from a minor and sinister solo to something fugal, finally soaring and ecstatic. (I dreamed of Kurt Weill.) Game as ever, Anita began bringing music the next day. At first almost liturgical, it otherwise had the spirit I'd imagined, and became lavishly complex by the end, to my astonished gratification. She gave the opening solo—set to a low reiterated minor line—to Charlotte to sing in her sharp, slightly heavy voice.

> *I couldn't run,*
> * I couldn't walk,*
> *I couldn't move,*
> * so I fled from the sun,*
> *Hugged me the dark,*
> * loved me the deep,*
> *Drank of my wound,*
> * ate of my heart,*

Feeling all ice
  bound to my wheel,
Forgetting to feel
  sitting alone
Gnawing my bone
Turning to stone
    to stone, stone

Then, after a piano interlude, Anita sings a kind of recitative describing Charlotte's encounter (lights should here come slowly up) with a group on wheels and on crutches (but also wearing goat's legs, birds' wings, animal masks in my dream production):

I groped in the dark and I stumbled and fell upon you
    and you and you and you and you and you and you and you
    and you!

Then, in major key Charlotte asks and Anita responds:

Give me a part,
  I'll take your part
My missing part
  I'll find you whole
No more apart
  We'll make a whole
How do we play
  This is the way

Here Jan, Wayne, Barry, and Ray come in with a plaintive line of equal beats:

A part to play each spinning day—

that they repeat throughout the now more rapid antiphony of Charlotte and Anita:

How do we play?
  This is the way
I'll take a part
  We'll make a whole
I can't walk
  We can dance
I can't run
  We can fly

What I miss
   We have found

Then while a diminished chorus repeats "A part to play each spinning day," others join Charlotte and Anita in triumphant and indeed soaring lines:

Give me a leg to stand on
   Get me up on your two feet,
You give me five,
   I'll lend you a hand

and now voices chase each other up the scale:

Leaning together we dance
Burning together we rise,
We'll pull the sun from its grave
   Make it run, make it fly
We'll pull the sun from its grave!

I'd half-forgotten my old flight fantasy until the song called it up—and illuminated it. I cannot speak for Ahab's tribe, but flight is my inevitable fantasy, for contradictory reasons. One I learned from being crippled: I've lost reliable contact with the ground—so how not dream of flying? I'd felt the other for that utopian moment in physical therapy; the workshop restored it as an ideal: I'm *more* grounded because more lodged in flesh, my body never again to be out of mind, and so—*potentially*—more whole, free, light.

The song made me happy because it captured so much of what I'd come to feel. But not all. On the last day before the rehearsal Barry offered an improv completely unlike his wild ghetto monologues. Tenderly mimicking man and child, he described his father teaching him to ride a bike. Pause. Then, in his own voice, "I was in the wrong place at the wrong time—and the wrong color." He'd been silent about his story and this miniature account surprised me into tears that, more surprise, I couldn't check. I had to leave the room. Barry's quiet piece had unleashed the sadness and loss at the base of all the valor, energy, and transcendence that so brilliantly displaced it.

The work-in-progress we presented after only nine days was a series of pieces. Each fragment was interesting and the whole was warmly received, but for various reasons the project went on ice.

"I prefer process," Joe had confided to us. "Final I don't like so much." At this writing, three years later, he still hopes to resume the project, but there are no funds, and other work calls. In two plays he directed recently, I saw Wayne perform. Charlotte and Ray are weathering the vicissitudes of acting in New York, and after retreating to Oklahoma, where he worked evenings with an amateur community theater, Jan has returned to New York to try his luck again.

Still working on his autobiographical musical, Barry is busy with his Déjà Vu company, his new DVC productions is about to launch a series of twelve performances integrating music, dance, theater, and fashion. He complained about the theater district's insensitivity to disabled members of the audience, insisting they sit in spaces from which "you need a telescope to see the stage." I told him that Kitty had mounted a demonstration on Easter Sunday at Radio City Music Hall to protest inadequate seating for viewers on wheels—and had won immediate concessions. She is studying dance again and teaching dance to children with disabilities who will "be mainstreamed into Jacques D'Amboise's National Dance Institute in May." Assailing many dance barriers at once, Kitty has started her own Infinity Dance Company—"the symbol of infinity is never-ending motion"—in which she dances in her chair along with two nondisabled male dancers over forty. Anita, who sometimes joins Kitty's company to sing, was recently nominated for a Helen Hayes Award for her performance in the musical play *The Fifth Season*. Anita plays a Dakota homesteader who loses her leg in the second act. Remarkably, the playwright and composer asked Anita to take the role because of her extraordinary voice without knowing she was an amputee. Recently Anita played a woman with polio in the New York reading of John Belluso's *Gretty Good Times*. She is currently touring with *Still Standing*.

As for me, I have retired early from teaching to struggle against (and adapt to) diminished strength—and to write my way through this adjustment. The work with the gallant creative crew in the Disability Workshop made it possible for me to start the transition to identification with my troubled body. Writing this piece helps me bear the reality that my adjustment is not complete and perhaps never will be. So it's a process—all I need now is, as Joe would say, to prefer it.

CONTRIBUTORS

Karen Alkalay-Gut teaches poetry at Tel Aviv University and chairs the Israel Association of Writers in English. Author of a biography of Adelaide Crapsey, she has also published fourteen volumes of poetry, including *The Love of Clothes and Nakedness* (Federation of Writers Union, 1999).

J. Quinn Brisben is a retired Chicago high school teacher who has been active in social causes since the 1950s and has been jailed eight times in the cause of disability rights.

Bell Gale Chevigny, recently retired from Purchase College, SUNY, published a revised and expanded edition of *The Woman and the Myth: Margaret Fuller's Life and Writings* (Northeastern University Press, 1994). She also published a novel, *Chloe and Olivia* (Grove Weidenfeld, 1990), as well as essays and fiction in many journals. She has been awarded a Soros Justice Fellowship for a project on prison writing and prison education.

Eli (Elizabeth) Clare is a poet, essayist, and activist living in Michigan. Her work has been published in a variety of periodicals as well as the anthology *The Disability Experience from the Inside Out*. Her book of essays, *Exile and Pride: Disability, Queerness, and Liberation*, appears from South End Press this year.

Susan Crutchfield is Assistant Professor of English at the University of Wisconsin at La Crosse, where she teaches cultural studies and film. Her article on representations of blindness in the slasher film appears in the collection *Mythologies of Violence in Postmodern Media* (Wayne State University Press, 1999), and she has an essay on the intersection of disability studies and film studies in *Disability Studies Quarterly* (Fall 1997). She continues to research and write on spectatorship and representations of blindness in popular cinema.

Mark DeFoe's third chapbook of poems, *Air,* appeared from Green Tower Press in 1998. He has poems forthcoming in *Monserrat Review, Rattapallax, Poet Love, Mangrove, Arkansas Review,* and elsewhere.

Stephen Dixon's nineteenth book of fiction, *Gould,* a novel, was published by Henry Holt in 1997. "The Motor Cart" is part of *Thirty*, an interconnected collection of fiction that is the sequel to *Gould;* it appeared from Holt in 1999. He teaches in the Writing Seminars of Johns Hopkins University.

Michael Downs received his MFA in fiction writing from the University of Arkansas's Programs in Creative Writing, where he was a Truman Capote Fellow. He teaches journalism at the University of Montana.

Marcy Epstein teaches English at Henry Ford Community College in Michigan. A Mellon fellow and recipient of the 1996 Neubacher Prize for the advancement of disability culture at the University of Michigan, she is the author of an essay on eating disorders and theatrical performance in *The Drama Review* (1996). She is currently at work on a book about disability and drama as well as a short memoir about her injury while in the West Bank in 1997.

Susan E. Fernback lives and writes in Berkeley, California. Her work has appeared in *The San Francisco Chronicle Sunday* and in *The Sun*.

Anne Ruggles Gere is Professor of English and Professor of Education at the University of Michigan where she directs the Joint Ph.D. Program in English and Education. She has published widely on composition studies, and her book *Intimate Practices: Literacy and Cultural Work in U.S. Women's Clubs 1880–1920* (University of Illinois Press, 1997) received the National Women's Studies Association Manuscript Prize.

Cynthia Margaret Gere studied painting at the Center for Creative Studies, the Institute for American Indian Art, and the University of Alaska at Fairbanks. With Anne Ruggles Gere, she is currently co-authoring *Woman of the King Salmon*, a book about life with Fetal Alcohol Syndrome.

Sandra M. Gilbert is Professor of English at the University of California, Davis. Her latest publications include *Wrongful Death: A Memoir* (W. W. Norton, 1995) and *Ghost Volcano: Poems* (W. W. Norton, 1995), as well as *The Norton Anthology of Literature by Women: The Traditions in English,* second edition (W. W. Norton, 1996), co-edited with Susan Gubar.

Joseph Grigely is an artist, critical theorist, and Associate Professor of Art at the University of Michigan. Among his recent exhibitions are solo shows at Galerie Francesca Pia, Bern; Air de Paris, Paris; the Anthony d'Offay Gallery, London; the MIT List Visual Arts Center; and the Douglas Hyde Gallery at Trinity College, Dublin. His publications include *Conversation Pieces* (Kitakyushu, CCA Kitakyushu, 1998),

Migrateurs (Paris, Musee d'art Moderne, 1996), *The Pleasure of Convers-ing* (London, Anthony d'Offay Gallery, 1996), and *Textualterity* (Ann Arbor, University of Michigan Press, 1995).

Brooke Horvath, an editor with the *Review of Contemporary Fiction*, teaches American literature at Kent State University. His most recent collection of poems is *Consolation at Ground Zero* (Eastern Washington University Press, 1995).

Georgina Kleege is the author of the novel, *Home for the Summer* (The Post-Apollo Press, 1989), and a book of personal essays about blindness, *Sight Unseen* (Yale University Press, 1999).

Victoria Ann Lewis is founder and director of OTHER VOICES, a program dedicated to new voices in the American theater, at Los Angeles' Mark Taper Forum. Her documentary plays and community projects include *Tell Them I'm A Mermaid* (1982), *P*H*reaks: the Hidden History of People with Disabilities* (1993), and the historic national gathering *A Contemporary Chautauqua: Performance and Disability* (1994). She is the co-author of *No More Stares*, and her articles have appeared in *Ms.*, *Disability Rag*, and *Spare Rib*. She is a Ph.D. candidate at the School of Theater, Film and Television at the University of California at Los Angeles.

David T. Mitchell teaches writing and American literature at Northern Michigan University. He is co-editor of *The Body and Physical Difference: Discourses of Disability* (University of Michigan Press, 1997), series editor of Corporealities: Discourses of Disability for the University of Michigan Press, co-founder and chair of the Modern Language Association's Disability Studies Discussion Group, and president of the Society for Disability Studies.

Carol Poore is Associate Professor of German at Brown University where she is introducing Disability Studies into the curriculum.

Burton Raffel has published poetry, fiction, and criticism in *MQR*. He has translated many authors into English, including Horace, Chairil Anwar, and Mandelstam. Most recently, his translations of five books by Chróetien de Troyes have appeared from Yale University Press.

F. D. Reeve is a poet and novelist whose recent books are this year's *The Moon and Other Failures* and 1995's *A Few Rounds of Old Maid and Other Stories*. He has received an Award in Literature from the American Academy of Arts and Letters and the New England Poetry Society's Golden Rose.

Sarah Ruden received her Ph.D. in Classics from Harvard and taught for several years in South Africa. (Her essay "Letter from South Africa" appeared in the Spring 1997 *MQR*.) Her book of poetry, *Other Places* (Jonathan Ball Publishers), won the 1995 CNA Award, the top South African book prize. She joined the Johns Hopkins University Writing Seminars in 1998.

Robyn Sarah is a Montreal writer whose most recent books are *Questions About the Stars* (1998), her sixth poetry collection, and *Promise of Shelter* (1997), a second volume of short stories. Her writing has appeared in *The Threepenny Review, New England Review, The Massachusetts Review,* and numerous anthologies.

Willa Schneberg's first book, *Box Poems,* was published by Alice James Books. Her poems have appeared or will appear in *Tikkun, Southern Poetry Review, Salmagundi, Double Take, American Poetry Review,* and the anthologies *Claiming the Spirit Within: A Sourcebook of Women's Poetry* (Beacon Press) and *Beyond Lament: Poets of the World Bearing Witness to the Holocaust* (Northwestern University Press). From 1992– 1993 she worked in Cambodia for the United Nations Transitional Authority. A photo-essay entitled "The Nuns of Monkol Won" appeared in the Spring 1998 issue of *Tricycle: The Buddhist Review.*

Reginald Shepherd's poem in this volume is from his third book, *Wrong* (University of Pittsburgh Press, 1999). The same press published his first two books, *Some Are Drowning* (1993 AWP Award) and *Angel, Interrupted* (1997 Lambda Literary Award finalist). He teaches at Cornell University.

Joan Seliger Sidney is the author of two poetry chapbooks, *The Way the Past Comes Back* (The Kutenai Press), and *Deep Between the Rocks* (Andrew Mountain Press). She leads writing workshops for both the Town of Mansfield and Windham Area Poetry Project.

Tobin Siebers, Professor of English at the University of Michigan, has published several books of literary criticism, most recently *The Subject and Other Subjects: On Ethical, Aesthetic, and Political Identity* (The University of Michigan Press, 1998) and *Cold War Criticism and the Politics of Skepticism* (Oxford, 1993). His collection of creative nonfiction, *Among Men,* appeared from the University of Nebraska Press in 1999.

Floyd Skloot's third novel, *The Open Door,* appeared in 1997 from Story Line Press, which will bring out his next collection of poetry, *The Evening Light,* in 2000. His essay on baseball and illness was included in *The Best American Essays 1993,* and his essay about his disabled brother's death will be included in *The Anchor Essay Annual/Best of 1999.*

Sharon L. Snyder teaches film and literature at Northern Michigan University. She is the co-editor of *The Body and Physical Differences: The Discourses of Disability* (University of Michigan Press, 1997), series editor of Corporealities: Discourses of Disability for the University of Michigan Press, and co-founder of the Modern Language Association's Disability Studies Discussion Group.

William Stafford's poem in this issue is one of the last he wrote. It appears in the posthumous collection *The Way It Is: New & Selected Poems* (Graywolf Press, 1998).

Rosemarie Garland Thomson is the author of *Extraordinary Bodies: Figuring Physical Disability in American Culture and Literature* (Columbia University Press, 1996) and the editor of *Freakery: Cultural Spectacles of the Extraordinary Body* (New York University Press, 1996). She is Associate Professor of English at Howard University in Washington, D.C.

Dallas Wiebe has won the Aga Khan Fiction Award from *Paris Review* and has been published in the Pushcart Awards volume. His novel *Skyblue the Badass* appeared in 1969 from Doubleday-Paris Review Editions, and Burning Deck Press has published three volumes of his short stories. His most recent book is a novel, *Our Asian Journey,* from MLR Editions Canada.